Laugh Your Way to Enlightenment!
The Art of Spiritual Laughter

Jessica Lloyd, Ph.D.

ISBN-13: 978-1519218025
ISBN-10: 1519218028

DEDICATION

To Mom

CONTENTS

ACKNOWLEDGMENTS

*In gratitude of those who have come before
and paved the way with laughter.*

> "THROUGHOUT THE CENTURIES
> THERE WERE MEN
> WHO TOOK FIRST STEPS
> DOWN NEW ROADS
> ARMED WITH NOTHING
> BUT THEIR OWN VISION."
>
> AYN RAND

"Only hyenas laugh"

-Mom

Only hyenas laugh,

Well... Hyenas and me.

I laugh.

In fact, I laugh a lot,

Much to my mother's chagrin.

You see, I'm not really supposed to be a laugher. In fact, I was raised to believe that only hyenas laugh. Children should be seen and not heard. Children should be quiet, behave, and be polite.

Of course, it didn't help that my natural laugh is more of a loud snort. You know the type that echoes in the room long after the joke has passed. Oh yeah, that's me... much to my mother's chagrin.

For me, childhood was serious business. Raised in a household where children were to be seen and not heard, laughter, silliness, and play eluded me. The house was quiet, respectful, and flawlessly operational. Saying please, thank you, and excuse me, were routine; laughing, however, was not.

So how does such a serious child discover the incredible power and freedom of laughter? Honestly, it wasn't easy... and it couldn't be simpler. My secret? Laughter Yoga. In March of 2014, I found myself at the Yogaville Satchidamanda Ashram near Charlottesville, VA attempting to become a Laugha (or Laughter) Yoga Leader. I was the only one there in blue jeans. My first clue, perhaps, that life as I knew it was about to change. A 6AM wake up call? No coffee? Vegetarian home-style meals? Umm... help.

Clearly, I had no idea what I was in for.

In fact, I'd signed up on a whim and had never seen or heard of Laugha Yoga before. But there I was, sitting in the beautiful Blue Ridge Mountains, watching in awe as Bharata Wingham, our Laugha Yoga Teacher, entered the room. He quietly sat on the floor and began to laugh. He laughed... and laughed. Why? For absolutely no reason at all!

My mother was right, he looked insane, but the light of his soul filled the room. I felt insane...

but I giggled. By the end of the course, I was hooked.

Those three days had changed my life. They cracked my shell - just a little - just enough to let a small ray of light in. You see, before arriving in Yogaville, I rarely laughed. It's not that I was depressed, I just didn't find that much to laugh about. Of course, I enjoyed a good Pixar flick and romantic comedies were high on my list, but beyond that... well... what can I say? Life was routine. Life was serious. Like so many of us, I'd focused on accomplishment and survival. And truth be told, as a single parent, I was far more likely to slip into tears than burst into laugher. And lets not forget, only hyenas laugh.

Upon leaving Yogaville, I vowed to bring more laughter into my life. I told my family and friends that I'd had a life changing experience. I posted it on Facebook. But like so many of us, my resolution to change gradually began to fade.
Life returned to normal; it became routine, and once again, rather serious. My beloved bursts of spontaneous laughter faded, and by August, they were gone.

Perhaps it was unrealistic to think that a child raised to be seen and not heard, would suddenly become an adult free to burst into uproarious laughter. Perhaps I expected too much from my three days with Bharta in Yogaville. Was my life changing epiphany simply the result of caffeine withdrawal? I have to admit, the idea haunted me. What had I experienced with laughter yoga? Was any of it real?

There was only one way to find out: I had to go back. So in August of 2014, I set off again for Yogaville. Though this time, I arrived prepared: This time I wore yoga pants and secretly packed my coffee pot.

The next three days flew by. I got up at 6AM. I ate vegetarian home-style meals, and most of all, I laughed. In fact, everyone laughed. We laughed until our sides ached. We snorted, we chuckled, we howled. We rolled on the floor and yes, my mother was right, we looked like hyenas. But once again, by the end of the weekend, I was hooked. Once again, I left Yogaville determined to change.

And this time; I did.

I joke now, telling my audiences that I failed the laughter yoga leader training course the first time around: That I am, perhaps, the only one in history to actually fail at laughing. But sadly I am not. In fact, laughter has long carried a stigma for adults.

Many of us have been socially conditioned not to laugh. We suppress our impulses and surrender our freedom. We've come to believe that we need justification for our laughter: If something is funny - I'll laugh. If nothing is funny - I wont laugh. Children laugh up to 300 times a day, but adults average only 7-12 laughs a day, (Altucher, 2014). And that's an average, meaning that some of us aren't laughing at all.

Many of us lose our capacity for joy as we

transition into adulthood. We forget how to play. We forget how to ignite our sense of wonder. Where we once looked at the world with awe - now we see annoyances. The grass in our front yard, for example, is no longer a welcomed invitation to walk bare foot or lie down staring up at the stars. Instead, the grass is a reminder of how there is never enough time in a day. It's too long... again. We see the bare spot - we see the weeds - next to our neighbor's perfection.

New discoveries and new experiences can also be met with distain. *"They changed Facebook again!"* we gripe to our friends. If the grocery store moves our favorite product, or construction reroutes our morning commute, our rhythm is shot. We feel off balance, un-happy, and confused. Far from the childlike wonder we once embraced, as adults we become creatures of habit. And few of us retain the habit of laughter.

Some, like my mother, genuinely believe that laughter is inappropriate, un-lady-like, or disruptive. Children should be seen and not heard: Ladies don't snort! In Japan it is considered rude to laugh without covering your mouth. Showing your teeth? How vulgar. In Turkey, Prime Minister Arnic recently declared it immoral for women to visibly laugh in public.

Perhaps he (and my mother) had gotten advice from Lord Chesterfield, who in the mid 1600s, stated:

> *"Observe it, the vulgar often laugh,*
> *but never smile, whereas well-bred*

people often smile, and seldom or never laugh. A witty thing never excited laughter, it pleases only the mind and never distorts the countenance."

Or St. Jean-Baptiste De La Salle, who wrote in *The Rules of Christian Decorum and Civility* of 1703:

"There are some people who raise their upper lip so high... that their teeth are almost entirely visible. This is entirely contradictory to decorum, which forbids you to allow your teeth to be uncovered, since nature gave us lips to conceal them."

As a result of these, and countless other examples, many of us have been socially conditioned not to laugh - at least not to laugh spontaneously.

Instead we seek out comedians and attend romantic comedies. We pay for our laughter. And even then, we do our best to laugh appropriately and for the right amount of time. We strive to laugh at the proper decibel. We laugh in groups - secretly hoping perhaps that our individual snorts and chuckles won't be singled out: That we, as Lord Chesterfield predicted, won't be the subject of ridicule.

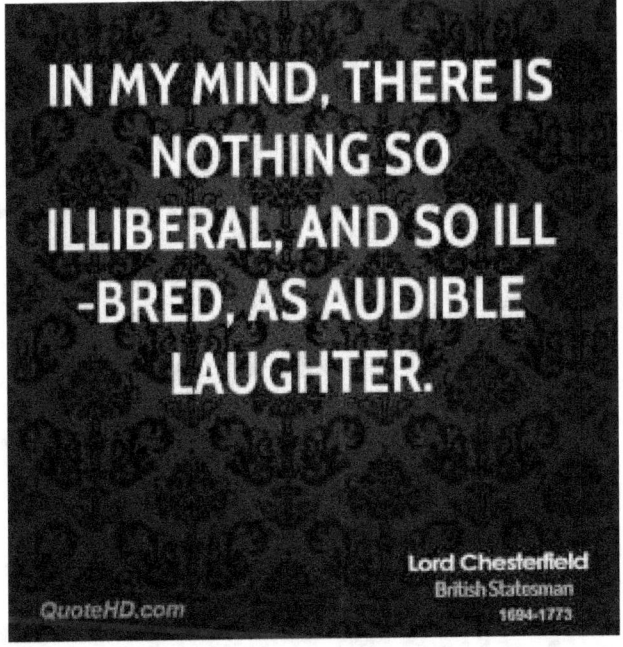

In short, we've given away our right and freedom to laugh, and as a result, laughter has become a valued commodity. But according to Bharata Wingham: *"There is not enough money in the world, to buy the amount of laughter America needs."* And I have to say, he might be right.

On August 4th 2009, USA Today declared that the number of American's using antidepressants has doubled in only a decade. In October of 2011, NPR reported that 1 in 10 Americans (or roughly 11% of the population) is currently taking antidepressants. Among women age 40-50, that number is 1 in 4!

The Mayo Clinic confers that the most commonly prescribed drugs in the United States today are antidepressants, but our underlying health problem is far larger. In fact, 70% of Americans take prescription drugs: Half of us are taking at least two medications, and one in five are taking five or more! (The Mayo Clinic, June 20, 2013) Clearly, we're paying for our laughter, or the lack there of, in more ways than one.

But what if I told you that you don't have to wait for something to make you laugh? That you don't need comedy, humor, or jokes? That you can chose to laugh your way back to health and happiness?

One just needs a little alertness to see and find out: Life is really a great cosmic laughter.

Osho

meetville.com

Many spiritual paradigms remind us that both joy and healing are within us. Buddhism teaches

8

that suffering is a choice. Christianity encourages us to surrender our troubles to God. The Bhagavad Gita states:

> *"When you experience things, like heat and cold, pleasure and pain, you only feel them because your senses are in contact with them. These things come and go. These things have the nature of impermanence, so watch them come and go with patience and an even mind."* (Srini, G. 2010).

In other words, while you may be unable to control or alter your experiences, you can choose how you react.

Are they right? Can we simply choose to be happy? Can we take back our innate control of joy and laughter? Can we laugh for no reason? Absolutely! Joy is our natural state.

Children play, explore, and embrace life. And most of all they laugh! They laugh until their sides ache: They roll on the floor. Even more astonishing, perhaps, is that children will laugh for absolutely no reason at all, something few adults retain the ability to do.... at least not before trying laughter yoga!

2. SO WHY AREN'T WE LAUGHING?

So why aren't we laughing? It seems easy enough. You simply open your mouth and laugh! Heck, babies do it: Children laugh 300 times a day. So what happens to adults? Why do we stop? Where does our laughter go? Are we secretly embracing the 16th century doctrine that laughter is vulgar? Do we still believe that covering our teeth at all times is paramount to our health?

Perhaps we're simply afraid to look foolish? Afraid that our smile lines and wrinkles will deepen? Perhaps we've seen a photo of ourselves while engaged in hearty laughter and realized that my mother was right, we do look like hyenas.

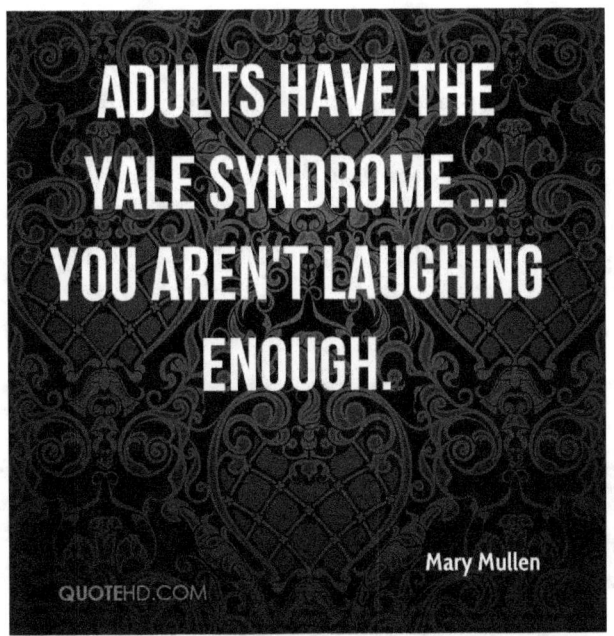

ADULTS HAVE THE YALE SYNDROME ... YOU AREN'T LAUGHING ENOUGH.

Mary Mullen

QUOTEHD.COM

Or maybe it's the sound of our laughter that stops us? Perhaps our laugh is too loud, funny, or downright embarrassing?   Truth be told, my laugh is embarrassing.   It's loud and awkward. While most people emit whatever laughter sounds they make as they exhale, mine comes on the inhale. It's as if I am desperately gasping for air while simultaneously say *hurp! "Hurp hurp, hurp", exhale, "hurp, hurp, hurp" exhale...* Needless to say, it isn't pretty. An introvert blessed with a loud rhythmic gasping style of laughter doesn't seem fair.   But for better or worse, my laugh immediately inspires more laughter around me: A fact I have long dreaded, and now embrace.

But alas, I doubt that laughter sounds, wrinkles, or 16th century beliefs, are what lies at the heart of why most adults stop laughing. In fact, I'd argue that the answer is far simpler and yes, even more obvious.

So why do adults stop laughing? Two words: Power and control. Mark Twain once said: *"Against the assault of laughter nothing can stand."* And I believe he's hit the nail on the head.

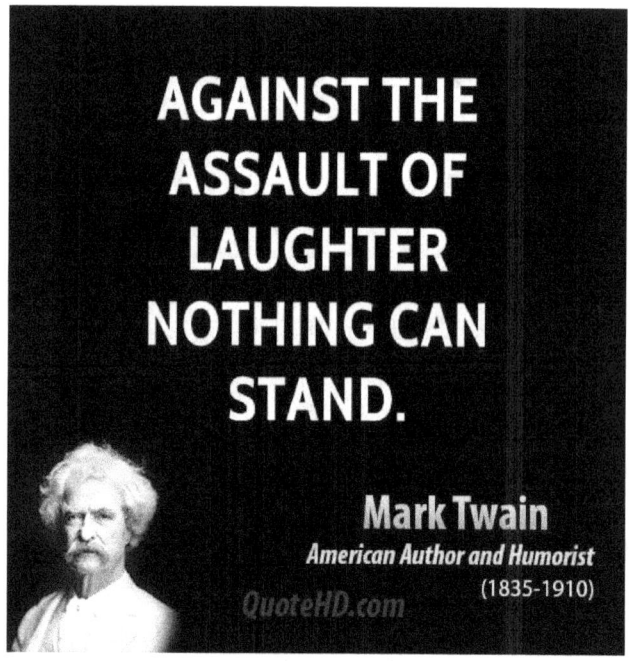

Think about it. Can you imagine the mayhem if laughter and play were free flowing in our public schools? What about our military? Our football teams? Our corporate offices and stores? If spontaneous laughter erupted 300 times a day among adults, it's no secret that nothing would get done.

Every teacher knows that once he or she loses a class to laughter, there is little hope of a quick recovery. Ever tried to scold a child who's laughing? It's not easy. Not only are you likely to end up laughing yourself, but even if you successfully retain your composure, you're bound to feel belittled or even mocked.

> One can never speak enough of the virtues, the dangers, the power of shared laughter.
>
> F. Sagan

Let's face it, laughter is disarming. It can be experienced as disrespectful, disempowering, and mean. Seriousness is thought to be a sign of honor and respect, while laughter is dangerous and rebellious. Laughing at a policeman, your boss, or a judge is clearly not a great idea. What if the United States military started laughing their way into combat? Would you still admire the bold and the brave? Imagine waiting to place an order in an expensive restraunt only to have your waiter arrive in the throws of laughter. Would you even attempt to continue with your order? What are the chances that you'd receive the correct meal?

Clearly we need at least some rules around laughter. I doubt anyone would argue in favor of a society based on constant uproarious chortles. Yet, I assert that our desire to control laughter runs deeper than social order, respect and productivity. In fact, I'd contend that its roots are deeply personal.

FEAR

I think people, on some level, are afraid of their own laughter. Why? Once again, the answer is likely power: Laughter renders us powerless. We can't control laughter, even when it's our own. There's no way to predict it. It comes without warning (or fails to show up when expected). Laughter can sneak up on us, catch us by surprise, and wreak havoc on our composure.

Lets face it, once it starts - I mean really starts -

we're simply powerless to stop it. Ever laugh at a funeral? In church? During a lecture? What happens when you tried to stop? Exactly! More laughter.

We all know that laughter is contagious. In fact, our brains are hardwired to respond to laughter with well... more laughter. Even the sound of our own laughter can stimulate us to continue.

Perhaps the most extreme example happened in 1962 when a small village in Tanzania, Africa experienced a *"Laughter Epidemic"*. It started on January 30th, 1962 with three young girls in a boarding school in Kashasha, Africa and spread, as laughter does, like wildfire. Approximately 60% of the school was quickly consumed by laughter. Symptoms of those affected lasted from a few hours to 16 days. The children's' behavior was so disruptive that the school was forced to close down, (Sebastian, S., 2003).

According to authorities, the epidemic quickly spread to neighboring villages. In April and May over 200 people had experienced long disruptive laughing attacks. By June, the epidemic had affected an additional 50 students in a neighboring school. In July, another outbreak occurred in the nearby village of Kanyangereka, and another two schools were closed.

By the end of the epidemic, 14 schools were shut down and over 1,000 people had been afflicted. To this day, scientists have no concrete explanation for what occurred in Tanzania. The general consensus is that the epidemic was the result of *Mass Psychogenic Illness* (MPI) brought on by mounting environmental and political stressors. A second, less recognized theory, claims its origins stem from a tainted food source, (Sebastian, S., 2003).

Though I doubt that any of us are afraid of a recurrent laughter epidemic, I do contend that laughing inappropriately carries such a negative social stigma that most of us secretly hope it won't happen to us.

Clearly laughter is powerful stuff. It breaks down walls, eliminates barriers, and draws people together. Laughter unites us. It bonds groups. It can disempower authority, disarm our defenses, and make us difficult to control.

PERSPECTIVE

There is one more reason we as a society seek to control laughter: *"Laughter can bring a new perspective"* (Christopher Durang). Laughter can inspire creatively, new thinking, new seeing. It threatens our cultural norms.

LAUGHTER CAN BRING A NEW PERSPECTIVE.

QUOTEHD.COM

Christopher Durang
American Playwright

Dr. Kataria writes:

> *"Laughter can't solve your problems, but it will dissolve them by changing your body chemistry and mindset so you can face them in a better way."*

It's no wonder perhaps, that we've sought to control our laughter. Personal and social change is always approached with trepidation, particularly change that has the potential to spread like wildfire.

If laughter has such a dark side - why embrace it at all. Why not simply be thankful that our children are ushered out of this free spirited danger zone and into a more serious world? Why would anyone want to look and sound like a hyena? Especially on a daily basis and for prolonged periods of time? The answer is simple: despite its occasional inconveniences, Laughter heals.

3. HEALTH BENEFITS

We've all heard it: Laughter is the best medicine. But few of us have any idea how true this is. Laughter offers a plethora of social, psychological and physical benefits and the list of continues to grow. Since Normand Cousins first reported healing himself through laughter after contracting a fatal disease in 1964, the health benefits of laughter, comedy and humor have peaked the interest of science.

Dr. Fry, (1994), of Stanford University, is credited with proving that laughter provides good physical exercise and lowers our risk of respiratory infections. He states:

> *"I believe that we do not laugh merely with our lungs, or chest muscles, or diaphragm, or as a result of a stimulation of our cardiovascular*

activity. I believe that we laugh with our whole physical being. I expect that this total participation will eventually be recognized."

He goes on to say,

" . . . it is appropriate to conclude that humor, mirth and laughter are on the side of contributing positively to the maintenance of health and survival, from the standpoint of their physiologic effects" (Fry, 1994).

Likewise, Dr. Berk, (1989), linked laughter to heart heath by studying its affect on arrhythmias, blood pressure, and recurrent heart attacks. Since then, the list of benefits associated with laughter has continued to grow.

Random Fact **#1848**

Laughter increases the activity of antibodies in the body by 20%, helping destroy viruses and tumor cells.

psychofactz.tumblr.com

Personally, I believe that nearly all of the health benefits associated laughter can be broken down in to two categories: Those that come from stress relief, basically allowing the body to *rest and reset,* and those associated with deep abdominal breathing.

Consider, for example, that laughing for 10 - 15 minutes a day can have the following affects on your body:

- Laughter lowers your stress levels by decreasing the cortisol levels in your body.
- Laughter increases serotonin levels in the body.
    - Releasing "feel good" chemicals in your brain, similar to a runner's high.
- Laughter helps regulate your blood sugar.
- Laughter lowers your blood pressure.
    - After experiencing an initial spike in blood pressure, a participant's blood pressure lowers and remains low for several hours.
- Laughter helps relieve pain.
    - After participating in 15 minutes of prolonged and sustained laughter, participants can experience up to 2 hours of pain relief.
- Laughter improves respiratory function.

- Encourages deep breathing
- Increases the oxygen available to your brain and body cells
- Laughter burns calories!
    - 15 minutes of hard laughter burns approximately 50 calories.
- Laughter exercises your facial muscles to give you a natural face-lift.
- Laughter boosts your immune system.
    - Raises T-cell production by stimulating the thymus glad to produce lymphocytes.
- Laughter exercises your internal abdominal muscles and provides a great abdominal workout.
- Laughter adds joy and zest to your life.
- Laughter decreases anxiety and fear.
- Laughter eases depression.
- Laughter improves your mood and enhances both emotional and physical resilience.
- Laughter makes you look younger.
- Laughter strengthens relationships.
- Laughter is attractive and draws others to us.
- Laughter promotes group bonding.
- Laughter breaks down walls between people.

HEARTY LAUGHTER IS A GOOD WAY TO JOG INTERNALLY WITHOUT HAVING TO GO OUTDOORS.

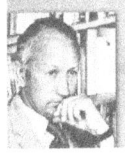

QUOTEHD.COM

Norman Cousins
American Journalist
1915 - 1990

Laughter can help regulate blood sugar? It lowers your blood pressure? Clearly laughing is a heart pumping exercise, but how does it lower (and not increase) your blood pressure? Likewise, at first glance, regulating blood sugar or blood pressure appears to have nothing to do with laughter... or does it?

As Dr. Frey (1994), states *"we laugh with our whole being,"* but perhaps this statement applies in more ways than one. Not only does laughter involve the entire physical body, it encompasses our *"psycho - social body" as well.*

RANGER

Several years ago, an animal control officer picked up a sad little dog in Austin Texas. The dog was mangy and flea bitten, his black and white fur - at least what was left of it, was matted and caked with mud. His deep brown eyes were filled with sorrow and fear. The little dog was brought in to the shelter, bathed, vetted and shaved. He placed in a large crate with warm blankets, fresh food and fresh water. The shelter employees named him Ranger and left him alone to eat.

Unfortunately, Ranger was terrified. Far from eating and rejoicing in his rescue, he sat shivering in the back corner of his cage. As the days passed, shelter employees became increasing concerned. Ranger was a pretty thin dog to begin with; not eating was not okay. The employees tried everything. Nothing worked. Until one day a volunteer mentioned that she had seen a program on PBS which discussed the concept of laughter and play among dogs. Within minutes, a plan was derived.

The volunteer went home and got out a tape recorder. For the next hour, she recorded the sounds of her own dogs panting and playing together. Happy healthy dogs, relaxed, well rested, well fed, and apparently producing the equivalent of dog laughter. She returned to the kennel and began to play back the recording for Ranger. Almost immediately upon hearing the sounds of the other dogs playing and "laughing,"

Ranger came to the front of the cage and began looking around. Within 10 minutes, he was eating. The kennel workers were thrilled. Yet in the mist of celebration, they noticed something else. The kennel was quiet! Not a single dog was barking. It was as if the recording had calmed not only Ranger, but everyone else in the room.

But why? There were already 20 - 25 dogs in the shelter, so it wasn't as if Ranger had been left alone. Likewise, the other dogs had been barking pretty regularly, why were they suddenly quiet? As it turns out, even listening to the sounds of laughter can have a calming effect on the body. And apparently, the same thing is true for dogs.

Why? Think about it, when do we laugh? We laugh when we're happy, well-rested and well-fed. We laugh with friends and family. We laugh when we feel safe. Ever been nervous about an important meeting or presentation only to have laughter lighten the load? The phrase comic relief stems from this phenomena. Laughter breaks through the tension and establishes a playful unity among people. It serves as a signal, perhaps to the most primitive parts of our brain, that we have come in peace - we are among friends. It's as if the laughter itself was saying to us: *Here, in this moment, you are safe.*

In today's 24/7 world, I'd venture to say the majority of us are racing through our days. We attempt to conquer a lengthy *To Do* list, constantly interrupted by email, texting, phone calls and snapchats. We are bombarded with advertising and marketing telling us that we need more energy, should move faster, be thinner, more beautiful and of course, get more done.

Facebook, Pintrest, and the Internet provide constant reminders of how much we miss while we sleep. Short video clips have replaced longer articles and emotionally charged protest fly with the click of a button.

Personally, I believe that at least half of the health benefits associated with laughter stem from its ability to interrupt our rushing. When we laugh - we stop - just for a moment, allowing our entire body to relax. We are not in the past, or in the future, we are simply here - present only in this moment. In that moment, we notice each other - we connect with those around us. Given its contagious nature, laughter can not help but to draw people together.

COMMUNITY

Laughter allows us to feel a part of something larger, and this too increases our sense of community, belongingness and joy. Dennis T. Jaffe, Ph. D., a Professor of Psychology at Saybrook Institute in San Francisco, found that "*A close-knit community can act as a protective envelope against stress.*" In other words, social interaction and networking are essential for happiness.

> # We also hope that a new type of industry will be created by linking the two different fields -- laughter and medical treatment.
>
> **Hikaru Horiguchi**
>
> QUOTEHD.COM

Likewise, numerous studies have suggested that people who possess a strong sense of community live longer. Those who feel valued, important, and able to affect the world around them simply live longer than those who don't.

We all want to be needed. We want to feel loved. But in today's fast paced world, many, particularly the elderly, are often over looked.

Families and friends move away, technology increasingly isolates us. Let's face it, in today's world there is little time for chatting with our neighbors.

> # A sense of humor... is needed armor. Joy in one's heart and some laughter on one's lips is a sign that the person down deep has a pretty good grasp of life.
>
> **Hugh Sidey**
> American Journalist

QUOTEHD.COM

But, laughter stops us, just for a minute. We *rest and reset* both physically and emotionally. We look up. We see each other; we see ourselves. Laughter provides an opportunity for the body to stop and recognize that it's safe. We laugh among friends. We laugh when we are healthy, happy, well rested, and well fed. We take a deep breath and calm down. Our biological systems are reset.

PAIN

Research shows that laughter decreases cortisol levels, essentially lowing the stress hormones in the body and increasing serotonin (the feel good chemical in our brain), (Berk, L.S. et al., 1989). In addition, the endorphins released during laughter provide a natural morphine affect. This allows a typical laughter session to provide up to two hours of pain relief without drugs. (Nasr, 2013). In other words, laughter does indeed allow the body to *rest and reset.*

DEPRESSION

Even more interesting perhaps is that this combination of decreased cortisol levels, increased serotonin levels, and the presence of a natural pain relieves, provides fertile ground to ward off depression. In fact, many who participate in regular laughter yoga sessions, report getting off their antidepressants, (Foley, et. al., 2002).

BREATH

Deep breathing is also important and responsible for many of the health benefits associated with prolonged laughter.

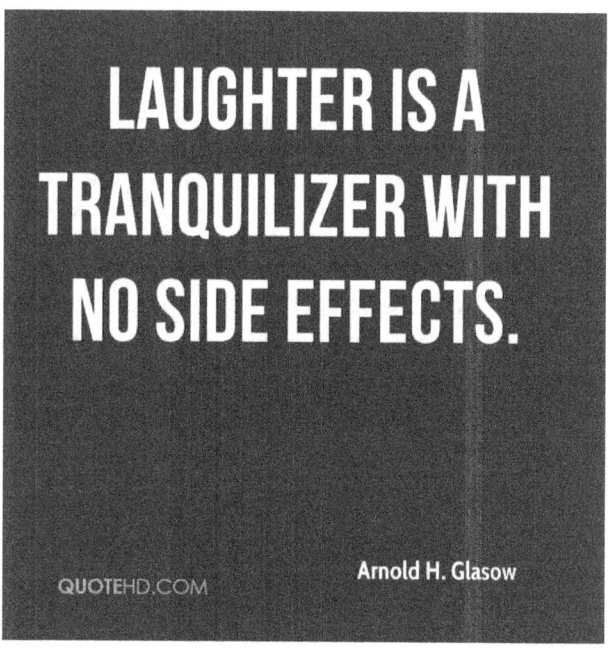

LAUGHTER IS A TRANQUILIZER WITH NO SIDE EFFECTS.

Arnold H. Glasow

QUOTEHD.COM

The breath is, in and of itself, a powerful healer. If you've ever laughed until your belly hurt, you're well aware that when you laugh you exhale deeply while engaging your abdominal muscles. Why does this matter? Consider the following:

The average male lung has a total capacity of about 6 liters of air. Yet as we sit in a resting state, watching TV or slumped over our computer, we typically breath in and out what is called the *Tidal Volume*, about 0.5 liters of air.   At rest this works for us, though it barely touches the full capacity of the lung.

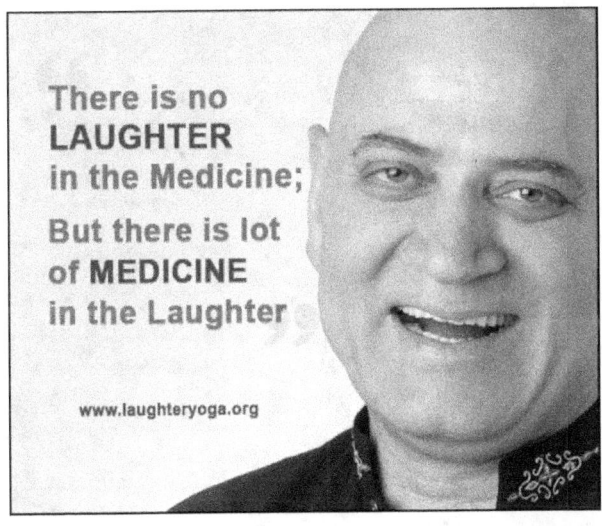

Another 1.5 liters of air, called *The Residual Volume*, remains in the lung at all times to keep it inflated. If you've ever experienced a punctured lung, collapsed lung, or had the wind knocked out of you, you know first had that losing this residual volume isn't fun.

But what happens in the doctor's office as a stethoscope is placed on your back?   As we're instructed to "take a deep breath," we take in about 2.5 liters of air, filling what is called the *Inspiratory Reserve Volume.* This process draws air into the upper chest, our shoulders rise as the rib cage rolls up and out. As you consciously inhale, you essentially fill this portion of your lungs.

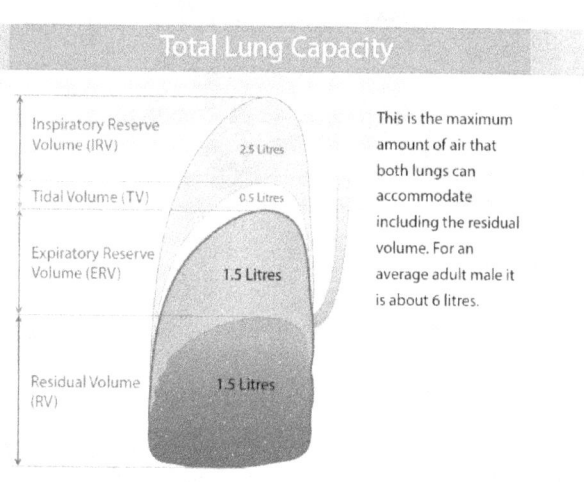

Total Lung Capacity

Inspiratory Reserve Volume (IRV) — 2.5 Litres

Tidal Volume (TV) — 0.5 Litres

Expiratory Reserve Volume (ERV) — 1.5 Litres

Residual Volume (RV) — 1.5 Litres

This is the maximum amount of air that both lungs can accommodate including the residual volume. For an average adult male it is about 6 litres.

Chart reprinted from: www.laughteryoga.org

Clearly we're moving a significant volume of air, engaging the potential of both the *Tidal Volume* and *Inspiratory Reserve Volume* of our lungs, but nearly 3 liters of our total capacity remains untouched.

In yoga and many other breathing practices, they refer to the three-part breath. This involves breathing sequentially into all three parts of the

lungs:
1. The abdomen (lower section of the lungs)
2. The ribcage
3. The chest

Students are instructed to begin by drawing the breath deep into the belly, feeling it rise with each inhalation and slowly fall with each exhalation.

The goal of *pranayama* breathing (or the yogic breath) is to exhale longer than you inhale. To begin, exhale by pulling the belly in towards the spine squeezing all that you can out of your lungs, as you release and begin to inhale, the belly will automatically rise drawing air deep into the base of the lungs, continue to inhale as you fill the ribcage and upper chest.

As you breathe from the diaphragm you tap into what is called the *Expiratory Reserve Volume*, and an additional 1.5 liters of air is exchanged. Because the act of laughing automatically engages the diaphragm and promotes extended exhalation, it too taps into the *Expiratory Reserve Volume*, and therefore, is considered a form of pranayama, or yogic breathing.

But why is this important?

Research has now shown that nearly all forms of cancer (and many other illnesses), are characterized by two basic conditions: acidosis and hypoxia (lack of oxygen) at the cellular level. In short, deep breathing may save your life.

Laughter affects the diaphragm, essentially engaging it and encouraging us to exhale deeply. Even to say: "*ha ha ha*" it becomes clear that with each sound the belly pulls in and the breath goes out. As we consciously exhale, we passively inhale to replace whatever volume of air was expressed. No doubt about it, the inhalation and exhalation of laughter clearly surpass the resting or tidal volume of air we would normally exchange, making more oxygen available to the body.

But taking in more oxygen and expelling carbon dioxide has another healing benefit: It shifts the body from an acidic to an alkaline state. Remember the two conditions associated with cancer: acidosis and hypoxia? Laughter eliminates both.

PH BALANCE

In recent years, countless books have been published promoting the idea of eating to balance the body's ph. Each claiming that we can eat our way to a more alkaline state and therefore remain cancer and illness free. While I have no comment on the validity of these works, I have purchased several of these books and have attempted to understand the countless charts and food categories described.

Eat this with this, but not that, and not alone. The rules seemed to go on and on! Foods I assumed were acidic, lemons and limes, for example, are actually basic, or at least produce an alkaline state in the body (Thom, M. & Wright, M.,

2013).

Needless to say, these charts are confusing and clearly it would be difficult to eat this way for long. But what if I told you that 10 to 15 minutes of laughter also shifts the body from an acidic to alkaline state? I don't know about you - but laughing seems a heck of a lot easier to me! As you laugh, you exhale while activating your diaphragm, forcing more carbon dioxide out of the body. As new oxygen rich air is drawn in, the pH of your body shifts from acidic to a more alkaline state.

Easy right? And don't forget that choosing laughter brings other health benefits as well. In fact, a seven year 54,000 person study concluded that people with a sense of humor have a 70% greater chance of surviving cancer, (Ellis, 2013).

Likewise, Norman Cousins, in his final book, *Head First: The Biology of Hope*, reported that 90% of the 649 oncologists he interviewed stated that an attitude of hope and optimism was the highest predictor of cancer survival.

Laugher also provides both stress and pain relief, something an alkaline diet can't even begin to do. In fact, I'd argue that attempting to alter your diet in such a dramatic way may in fact cause you more stress. (Not that such diets are not beneficial, I have no doubt that they are, but for the sake of comparison, laughter wins hands down as the easier route.)

LAUGHTER IS BY DEFINITION HEALTHY.

Doris Lessing
Persian Novelist

QUOTEHD.COM

Balance Your pH Food Chart example:

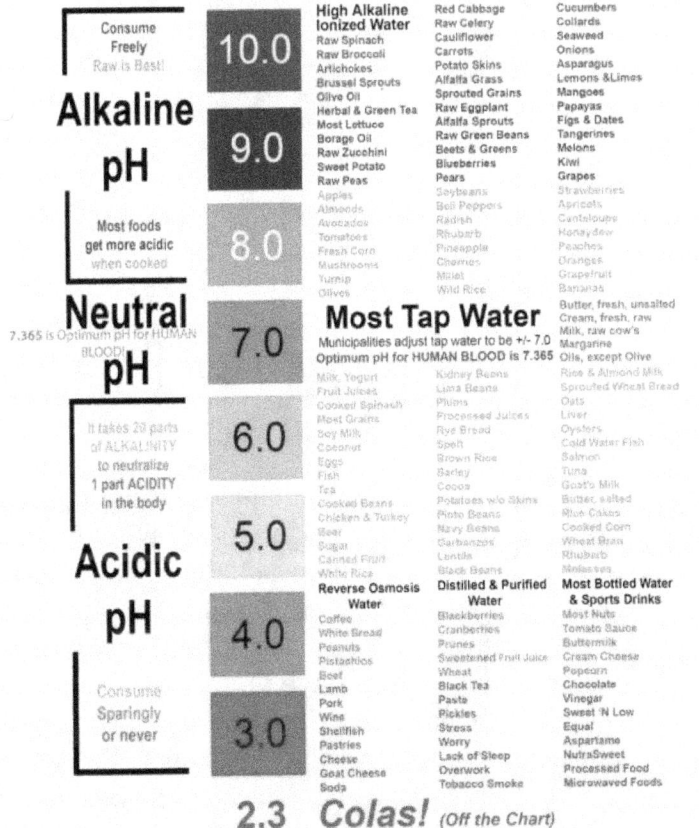

(Image source: http://alkalinejourney.com)

(Notice that colas are so acidic they are not even included in the "food and beverage" realm.)

4. LAUGHTER YOGA:
TAKE BACK YOUR LAUGH

Sadly, it seems many adults lose their ability to laugh, or at best, are laughing an average of 12 times a day. Some, like myself, have never found their laugh to begin with. Others, perhaps, have simply forgotten how to laugh. Maybe we're too stressed, too tired, or have too many deadlines to meet. Perhaps the desire for spontaneous chuckles has been socialized away. Yet where ever your laughter went, you can get it back!

Laughter yoga allows adults to rekindle the sense of freedom they had as children to laugh and play. It encourages us to break the cycle of cause and effect laughter. It teaches us to laugh pro-actively rather than re-actively. Because the truth is, you don't need others to make you laugh. You don't need comedy or jokes, in fact, it's more empowering if you don't have them. Everything you need to be happy is within you. How do you access it? The answer is easy: just laugh!

THE CHILDLIKE PHYSICALITY OF LAUGHTER EXERCISES IS RESTORATIVE FOR ADULTS.

Steve Wilson

I know it sounds crazy, don't forget, I had to go to Yogaville twice before I believed it myself. Perhaps you're sitting there thinking, but how can you laugh for no reason? Managing a small chuckle is one thing, but to laugh? Really laugh? For absolutely no reason at all? Without comedy, humor or jokes? That's ridiculous.

You're right. I completely agree. It is ridiculous, but it's also sheer brilliance. In laughter yoga we simply *fake it until we make it* which honestly, when you're laughing in a group takes all of about 30 seconds. If laughter tells the brain that it's happy - and you want to be happy - then... well... laugh!

> # In Laughter Yoga,
> # "We don't laugh
> # because we are happy;
> # we are happy
> # because we laugh"
>
> ### - Dr Madan Kataria

Laughter yoga is based on the belief that voluntary laughter provides the same social, psychological and physical benefits as spontaneous laughter. Just as we exercise our physical bodies by lifting weights or using a treadmill, we can exercise our laughter. To do so, you simply practice laughing. You laugh frequently and for no reason at all. In essence, you fake it until you make it.

You may feel silly, especially if you, like me,

have been raised not to laugh, but remember medical research has proven it works. In fact, according to Neuro Linguistic Programming (NLP) there is little difference between thinking about doing something and actually doing it. (A fact most pro ball coaches and players have known for years.)

> *"Where thoughts lead, chemicals follow"*
>
> -Deepak Chopra

Still not convinced? Remember Ivan Pavlov? Ivan was a Russian scientist, awarded the Noble Prize in 1904 for his research on operant conditioning. Ivan demonstrated that after consistently ringing a bell before feeding his dogs, the dogs quickly began to anticipate eating upon hearing the bell - even with no food in sight. Their reaction was obvious: the sound of the bell triggered thoughts of food and produced drool. Try it. Think of your favorite food... a warm chocolate chip cookie, a ripe peach, hot apple pie: Getting hungry? Can you taste it? Smell it, almost see it there before you? Is your mouth watering?

Mine is.

Actors are well aware of this principle. Need to look sad in a movie? No problem, just think about being sad... remember sad times... make sad faces and pretend to cry.

Sexual arousal is no different and the advertising industry is counting on it. Want to feel better about yourself? Buy the car with the beautiful model draped over it. In other words, fake it until you make it!

When you laugh
or smile, it
triggers
a part of your
brain that actually
makes you Happy

Unfortunately the benefits of laughter on the body don't show up as quickly as dog's drool. In fact, the social, psychological and physical benefits of laughter require three things: 1) The laughter must be prolonged and sustained (a 10-

15 minute session), 2) It must be a deep belly laugh (coming from the diaphragm) and 3) A daily laughter practice is necessary to sustain results.

Sadly, most adults don't have the opportunity to experience periods of prolonged or sustained laughter. In fact, natural laughter (if and when it occurs) tends to last only a few seconds, not enough time to bring about the desired biochemical changes.

Likewise, we are not naturally prone to engage in deep belly laughter. Socially conditioned to laugh quietly (or not at all), many of us hold back. Too self conscious, or trapped in an environment where prolonged laughter might be considered inappropriate, we are lucky to experience a quiet chuckle once or twice a day.

In addition, most of us have relinquished control of our laughter. By waiting for something funny to happen before we laugh, we've become dependent on others, dependent on external stimuli, and left to seek out comedians and / or doctors to stay healthy. Laughter yoga allows us to stop leaving our laughter to chance. We can take back our personal power and control of our laughter. Like any other form of exercise, we can laugh, at any time, for any reason - or for no reason at all.

ORIGINS OF LAUGHTER YOGA

Laughter yoga was started by Dr. Madan Kataria in Mumbai India. Though his work in the medical field, Dr. Kataria had become increasingly aware of the health and healing benefits of laughter. So on March 13th 1995, he gathered his wife, Madhuri and three friends in a public park to laugh together.

Initially the participants took turns telling jokes or sharing funny stories. The group quickly grew and within two weeks they had over 50 members. Unfortunately, they also had a problem. The flow of good jokes and happy stories had been exhausted. Hurtful, negative and offensive jokes began to emerge. Several members were insulted and began to complain.

Dr. Kataria was desperate for a solution. He quickly found it in the literature: The human body cannot tell the difference between real and fake laughter.

Both produce the same beneficial effects. Armed with this information, he returned to the club. This time encouraging members to laugh for no reason. To spite their initial skepticism, club members soon found themselves laughing like never before.

Dr. Kataria went on to develop a wide range of laughter games and exercises which have now been taught all over the world.

His wife, Madhuri, a yoga instructor and the Co-founder of Laughter Yoga incorporated the many yogic breathing and Pranayama exercises, and Laughter Yoga was born.

Excerpt from: *Laugh for No Reason*, by Madain Karatia

BUT WHAT'S WRONG WITH JOKES?

Absolutely nothing! Jokes are wonderful! Comedy is incredible, silly stories - bring them on! Don't forget, Norman Cousins cured himself by watching funny movies. In fact, a great deal of the research done on the health benefits of laughter has employed comedy (funny videos, jokes, stand up comedians, etc.) as the delivery method.

But humor is a tricky thing. For starters, it's dependent on both internal and external stimulus. It requires both a trigger and a response. It depends on you and a source. Humor is actually a three step process. In other words, first something funny must happen, then you perceive the event as funny, and finally, you laugh. Your experience, your environment, your mood, even your cognitive function will play a role in the outcome.

Ever heard a wonderful joke that was delivered poorly? Have a friend who consistently screws up the punch line? What if you don't feel like laughing? You're depressed, grumpy or angry, and nothing seems funny? Or perhaps you simply don't understand the punch line?

Humor is a culturally dependent construct. It relies heavily on cognitive function and is context and environment specific. A plumber, for example, may not understand an electrician's favorite joke and vice versa. Let's face it, jokes often fall flat. Thus, trusting your health to humor stimulated laughter is a risky business. You may laugh, but you may not.

For the sake of argument, let's say that you do laugh. You're at a party: You feel happy and are healthy, when the joke is told. You laugh, the crowd laughs, yay! Yet, because adults use cognitive function to comprehend humor, humor stimulated laughter, even when effective, remains a mental exercise. Remember humor is a three step process: someone tells a joke, we understand the joke, then we laugh. Yet anytime you engage the brain to promote understanding, judgment and social constraint also engage.

How much should I laugh? How long can I laugh without looking foolish? Is anyone watching? Are they laughing too? Good grief, what would Lord Chesterfield think? For better or worse, once we begin laughing, we quickly become conscious of others around us. We strive to fit in, to laugh appropriately. Given that 10 - 15 minutes of prolonged and sustained deep belly laughter are necessary for the health benefits to engage, the *humor model* of laughter is clearly limited.

"When your happiness
is dependent upon
what is happening
outside of you,
constantly you live
as a slave to the
external situation."
— Sadhguru

Rarely do adults laugh for more than a few seconds after hearing a joke. Even a full minute of laughter would likely prove awkward in a social setting. Laugh for a full minute after hearing a joke, and your friends and family will think you've lost your mind.

Children, on the other hand, laugh from their hearts. They laugh for no reason at all. A child's laughter stem from silliness and play. They require no external stimulus. There are no jokes to comprehend and no sense of humor is required. Their laughter simply flows. This model of humor is called the *Childlike model* or

Body-to-Mind model and is what laughter yoga strives to employ.

Because intellectual processing and cultural understanding are not required, childlike laughter is not limited to healthy individuals or those with good cognitive functioning. Language barriers are dissolved. Age, intellectual comprehension and even dementia disappear as constraints. Without engaging the mind, the laughter flows easily. There is no room for judgment; no need for thought. Laugher comes easily and the vast array of health benefits stemming from prolonged and sustained laughter emerge.

ETHICS OF LAUGHTER

It's important to remember that laughter, particularly when it comes in the form of jokes and comedy, can be used as a tool, or as a weapon.

Laughter yoga, in its utilization of childlike playfulness and underlying principle of laughing for no reason at all, seeks to eliminate all hostile, critical or sarcastic humor. By laughing as a physical exercise and for no specific reason, laughter yoga participants consciously avoid resorting to ridicule, rude, inappropriate or offensives approaches to humor.

5. WHY IS IT CALLED YOGA?

The word yoga comes from the Sanskrit root "yuji" meaning to link or connect, to draw together or harmonize. Yoga is about integration and balance. Linking the body and breath. It's about being connected, being aware and being aligned with yourself.

The simple process of laughing draws us into the present moment. You cannot laugh in the past or future; laughter resides only in the here and now. When we laugh, we are completely engaged and absorbed in the experience. When we laugh we let go of our egos and embrace our hearts. Unconditional laughter can awaken your capacity for unconditional love. In short, laughter links us - not only to others, but also to ourselves.

Aside from the wonderful physical benefits of laughter, establishing a regular laughter practice can provide the space necessary for our true nature to emerge. Laughter stops us in our tracks and disrupts, even if just for a moment, the organized chaos of our lives. In other words, yogic laughter enables us to lose ourselves - in order to find our true and higher selves.

Through laughter, we break our routines. We create space. We let go of chronic seriousness; let go of tension, routines, and control. We let go of ego. Through laughter, we manifest a type of emptiness - a space - a freedom perhaps, into which our true selves can immerge. In short, intentional yogic laughter shorten not only the distance between our self and others, but even more importantly it shortens the distance between our self and our higher self.

No doubt you've notice the effects of laughter on a group? How quickly tension is dissolved? How quickly egos and power are equalized? Yet few of us recognize this process occurring within ourselves. Just as laughter serves to create an more balanced playing field within a group, it serves to create a unity or equality among all parts of an individual. Are you stress levels sky rocketing? Tension, fear, anger, out of control? Feeling depressed and frustrated? Want everything to return to a more balanced state? The answer is easy: Laugh!

> "Laughter Yoga combines laughter with yoga breathing exercises. It is a perfect way to laugh and get exercise at the same time. It approaches laughter as a body exercise so it's easy to laugh even if you're depressed or in a bad mood. I've tried it, and it works."
>
> - Oprah Winfrey

Likewise, laughter yoga links the body and breath and incorporates many aspects of *Pranayama*, the ancient practice of yogic breathing. *Prana, or life force energy*, is believed to enter the body through the breath. As we become stressed our breathing becomes shallow, and the flow of *Prana* diminishes.

The main characteristic of all yogic breathing exercises is that the exhalation be longer than the inhalation.   This is indeed the case with many laughter yoga exercises.   Even the act of saying "*ha, ha, ho, ho*" is an exercise in exhalation.   In this sense laughter yoga is appropriately named.

Laughing is, and will always be, the best form of therapy.

AUTHOR
DAU VOIRE

6. THE POWER OF THE
BREATH AND BODY CONNECTION

Laughter has a super power. Well, truth be told, all breathing exercise do, but laughter is by far the easiest and the most enjoyable way to activate the magic.

Let me explain. The human body is an intricate system regulated predominately by the brain and central nervous system. (Of course, the heart plays a huge role, but for the sake of argument, let's focus on the brain.) In this analogy, let's say the brain is serving as CEO of the body. Serving under the CEO are two branch managers: the *sympathetic nervous system* and the *para-sympathetic nervous system.*

Now these two divisions operate and cooperate with a tag team style of management. Though they work side-by-side, happily carrying out their individual duties, they pass their dominance, or leadership responsibilities, back and forth. Like cyclists drafting each other in a race, the sympathetic and parasympathetic nervous systems pedal along side by side, as they jockey for the lead.

The *parasympathetic nervous system* is a fairly relaxed manager. Not in any particular hurry, this system is responsible for regulating the body's resting state. Known as the *feed and breed* or *rest and digest* system. The parasympathetic system helps regulate gastric juices, bowel function, resting heart rate and blood pressure. It monitors kidney function, sexual function, etc. Overall a pretty laid back manager, concerned primarily with making sure everyone shows up on time and preforms their routine duties.

The *sympathetic nervous system* however, has more of a type A personality. This system is reactive, up tight and high strung. Known for its *fight or flight* response, the sympathetic nervous system is responsible for our state of arousal. It has *sympathy* for our condition and reacts to protect or defend us. It gets us moving. Like a child throwing a temper tantrum, the sympathetic nervous system demands to be noticed. It shuts down unnecessary bodily functions, shunts blood away from the kidneys and GI tract. Our heart rate and blood pressure increase, our pupils dilate, we begin to sweat and are ready to run, fight, or flee. Not unlike the screaming child, you can't ignore or easily calm the sympathetic nervous system.

There is however, something that works: A magic bullet or pacifier, if you will. Both systems share a common element. They both regulate the breath.   When the parasympathetic system engages, the breath is calm and steady. We're relaxed, resting and digesting. Engage the sympathetic system and the breath becomes rapid - we're alarmed and ready to fight or flee. Yet this shared control of the breath - or more specifically the diaphragm, provides the brain with an over-ride switch.

When the sympathetic system engages unnecessarily, for example, when we're stressed at work or nervous about a presentation, we can over-ride this biological fight or flight response by consciously engaging the diaphragm. As you breath deeply, activating the diaphragm,   you signal the parasympathetic nervous system to take the lead. As soon as it does, the body begins to shift back to a more relaxed state.

So what does this have to do with laughter? Laughter engages the diaphragm. It encourages us to breath deeply, exhale fully and from the belly. In short, laughter shifts us from a state of alarm, stress, and shallow breathing to a state of relaxed, calm, deep breathing.

People who laugh actually
live longer than those
who don't laugh. Few persons
realize that health actually
varies according to the
amount of
laughter.
-James J. Walsh

The diaphragm is the only known element in the human body that is both consciously and unconsciously regulated. Think about it. You can't consciously control the speed of your GI track - you can't consciously regulate your kidney function, nor can you consciously regulate your blood pressure or heart rate. Sure, a trained practitioner can lower their heart rate through meditation, but guess how they do it? Exactly - they engage the diaphragm.

Through taking long deep breaths, slowing the breath, and pausing gently between breaths, an experienced yogi or meditator can indeed lower their heart rate. But they aren't directly effecting the heart. We can't simply command our heart rate or blood pressure to decrease. But we can engage the parasympathetic nervous system: By consciously activating the diaphragm, taking long, slow, deep breaths, exhaling fully - or simply laughing, we can over ride the sympathetic nervous system. Control of the body temporarily returns to the parasympathetic branch and a more restful state ensures.

WHAT DO I NEED TO BRING?

Nothing.

A yoga mat? Nope.
Special shoes? Nope.
Special clothes? Nope.
Expensive gear? Nope.

A sense of humor? Nope.
Good mood? Nope.
Healthy body? Nope.

Do I need:

To be able to do yoga? Nope.
Able to walk? Nope.
Able to stand? Nope.

The truth is, all you have to do is show up. In fact, recent research shows that even listening to laughter can have positive benefits on your health. (Adorn Journal, 2004).

7. THE MAGIC INGREDENTS: FOUR ELEMENTS THAT MAKE IT WORK

There are four key elements, or components of laughter yoga that seem to make it work. In fact, it works so well, Dr. Kataria has been conducting laughter yoga sessions with prison inmates all over Mumbai, India. Talk about a tough crowd!

The magical combination of these four elements: eye contact, clapping, laughing, and playfulness, ensures that you don't need a sense of humor to laugh. You don't need to be in a good mood, in fact, you don't have to feel like laughing at all. When these elements come together, it simply becomes hard not to laugh.

EYE CONTACT

Laughter yoga participants are encouraged to

make eye contact with each and every person they encounter during a session. On the surface, this element simply makes the whole experience funnier. Lets face it, if you're being silly and you see someone else being silly, you're bound to feel even more ridiculous! Likewise, if you start laughing, the person you're looking at will soon follow. You look around, they look around, and trust me, soon everyone is laughing. Remember the Laughter Epidemic of 1962 in Tanzania? Laughter is contagious!

But the presence of eye contact plays another important role in making laughter yoga unique. It has a subtle, but very important, function. In society today, it seems that no one sees each other. I mean really sees each other. People are rushing around here and there. We're on our phones, at the computer, in our cars. We send email and text messages rather than meeting face to face. We communicate through Facebook and Twitter, constraining our lives into a 140 character allotment. Snapchat messages and images disappear in under 10 seconds. We hear stories of people being trampled during a Black Friday sale. The homeless are passed by: the elderly overlooked. Let's face it, opportunities to make meaningful eye contact are not what they used to be, and in many ways, it's only getting worse.

There was a story floating around Facebook a while back about a baby dolphin who had washed up on the shore at a popular resort location.

Beachgoers found the adorable creature and a crowd gathered. Before long they began taking selfies with him. Holding the dolphin and smiling brightly, the beachgoers eagerly passed him from person to person: The dolphin died. Of course, no one intended to harm the little guy. In fact, they thought he was adorable. Yet despite everyone looking at him. no one actually *saw* the dolphin. Why? Because looking and seeing are not the same thing.

I contend that we've turned into a society that simply looks. We look past: We look through, but rarely do we see each other. Like the beach going tourist, with cell phone in hand, we see the shape and basic configuration of life, but we fail to see its condition. We recognize an adorable baby dolphin; but fail to see it grasping for air.

But in laughter yoga we do see each other. We look each other in the eye and amazing things happen. Not only do we burst out laughing, but communities and friendships are formed. We learn each other's names. We check on each other, care about each other, and most of all, we laugh.

CLAPPING

In laughter yoga we clap with a flat hand in a large exaggerated way. This style of clapping is two fold. First, there are a lot of energy centers and nerve ending in the palms of the hand and fingertips. Clapping with a flat hand serves to stimulate these centers. It also makes you feel silly. Large exaggerated clapping is more childlike - more invigorating and simply more fun.

BREATHING / LAUGHING

Talk about health benefits! Laughter yoga is called yoga because of its incorporation of *pranayama*, or yogic breath. In short, laughter causes you to exhale fully and from the diaphragm. As we laugh or simply say *Ha Ha - Ho Ho* during a laughter yoga session, we naturally exhale deeply. Pulling the belly in and activating the diaphragm increases the amount of oxygen available to our bodies and shifts our pH balance to a more alkaline state. And don't forget, research has shown that nearly all forms of cancer (and many other illnesses), are characterized by two basic conditions: acidosis and hypoxia (lack of oxygen) at the cellular level, (Young & Redford Young, 2002). In short, laughter, or more accurately, the deep breathing associated with laughter, may add years to your life.

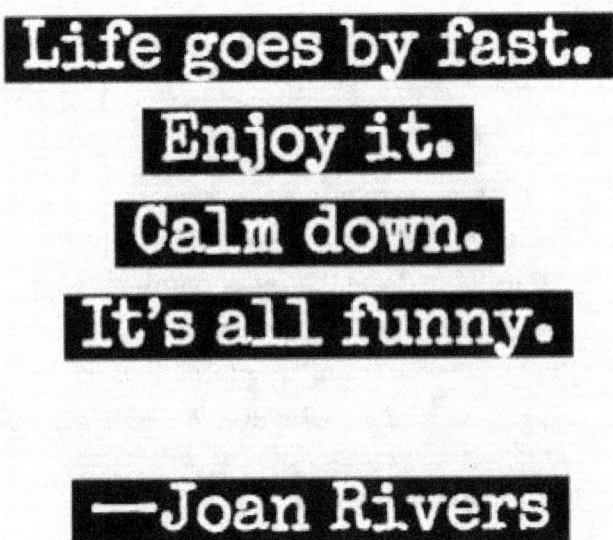

**Life goes by fast.
Enjoy it.
Calm down.
It's all funny.**

—Joan Rivers

PLAYFULNESS

For many, this may be the hardest element of laughter yoga to embrace. But spontaneous laughter and playfulness are intimately connected. If you begin to play - you will begin to laugh. You become happier. You draw in a new sense of creativity and fun. Suddenly things which never seemed funny before will have you in stitches. In short, play helps adults lighten up. We let go, just a little, just enough to let the laughter flow.

Osho, a 20th century spiritual leader, teacher and philosopher writes:

> *"Playfulness is one of the most repressed parts of human beings. All societies, cultures, civilizations have been against playfulness because the playful person is never serious. And unless a person is serious he cannot be dominated, he cannot be made ambitious, he cannot be made to desire power, money and prestige."*

He goes on to state:

> *"Society is always afraid of non-serious people."*

Both Osho and Dr. Kataria believe that play will arouse laughter and perhaps more importantly, that laughter destroys "*headiness*" or ego. As we shift our attention to play, our focus shifts to the heart. Osho contends that it is seriousness that causes wars, seriousness that causes stress and disease in the body. Yet laughter and play awaken our joy and bring more life to our beings.

By drawing these four elements together, *eye contact, clapping, breathing / laughing,* and *playfulness*, laughter yoga participants quickly turn forced laughter into real laughter. Our inner-children awake, seriousness dissolves, and joy bubbles up inside of us.

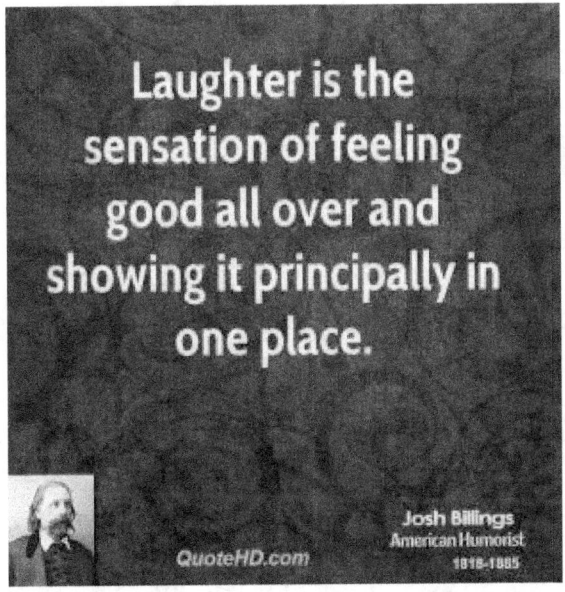

Laughter is the sensation of feeling good all over and showing it principally in one place.

Josh Billings
American Humorist
1818-1885

QuoteHD.com

8. STUMBLING INTO JOY!

Seek joy not happiness. Umm, okay. But what exactly does that mean? What is joy anyway? How is it different than happiness? And more importantly, why do we care?

Honestly, before I discovered laughter yoga, the constructs of joy and happiness were simple abstractions. Flooded with magazine and television ads, I, like so many others, sought to find happiness in the external realm. I made lists, embarrassingly long lists, of what was required to ensure my happiness. To be happy, I decided, meant to achieve, not only materially but also educationally, socially, and personally. So off I went in pursuit of these goals. I acquired a college degree, a husband and a child - sure I'd found the winning combination for happiness. But indeed, I had not. Hmm... perhaps a master's degree? Another child? A new house, new car, new job?

Perhaps I should run a half-marathon? Lose weight? Or dress differently? Three children, a PhD, 12 half-marathons, and countless wardrobe changes later, yet, I had failed to secure happiness.

> *The most beautiful moments in life are moments when you are expressing your joy, not when you are seeking it.*
>
> ~ Sadhguru Jaggi Vasudev ~
>
> OkyDay.com

HAPPINESS

So what is happiness anyway? And why is it so hard to find. According to Google, happiness is the state of being happy. Not a definition I found particularly helpful. Ironically, Google goes on to supply the following sentence: *"She struggled to find happiness in her life."* Talk about a sense of humor! Seems even Google dictionary is struggling to define this term.

The Webster Dictionary however, offers slightly more. According to Webster: Happiness is synonymous with the terms: good fortune and prosperity. The following sentence is provided: *"Her happiness was complete when she got her own house."* Again rather ironic, as I had a house, a big house in fact, could I too say my happiness was complete?

Clearly, the construct of happiness is linked to obtainment. It carries an if / then statement. If I get this - then I'll be happy. If I achieve this - then I'll be happy. If I look like this, buy this, go here, then I'll be happy. Talk about an advertiser's dream come true! Unfortunately, this model of happiness leaves us in a never ending cycle. Happiness is always moving. It's a goal we can never fully obtain. If a college degree didn't ensure my happiness, perhaps a master's degree would? Still not happy? Clearly a PhD is required. It seems it never ends. Even the declaration of independence refers to the PURSUIT of happiness, not its attainment.

LET THERE BE MORE JOY AND LAUGHTER IN YOUR LIVING.

QUOTEHD.COM

Eileen Caddy
English Celebrity

JOY

Joy however, is a different story. Where happiness comes from the head - joy comes from the heart. Joy is an emotion. It stems from well-being and contentment. Webster Dictionary gives the following sentences as examples of joy:

"Their sorrow turned to joy"

"I can hardly express the joy I felt at seeing her again."
"The flowers are a joy to behold."

See any stuff in there? Anything to buy? To obtain? To accomplish? Exactly. Joy is unconditional. Joy comes from the heart. And joy, unlike happiness, is directly linked to laughter.

If we shift our emphasis away from happiness and towards seeking joy - seeking the emotion of well-being and contentment, happiness will inevitably follow. Just as the presence of play evokes laughter; the presence of joy evokes happiness.

9. LAUGHTER AS A SPRIRITUAL PRCTICE

Dr. Kataria, the founder of the Laughter Yoga movement, has gone out of his way to ensure that laugher yoga is not associated with any particular religious doctrine. It is his vision that everyone be welcomed at all times, in all countries, all cultures and languages. Yet, Dr. Kataria also readily admits that laughter yoga stems far beyond simply laughing.

He writes:

> *Laughter yoga goes beyond just laughing. It not only fosters a feeling of physical well being, it enhances the spirit and touches the emotional core. It cultivates positive thinking and*

promotes understanding. Many of the laughter exercises focus on forgiveness, generosity, compassion, and helpfulness. Laughter Yoga gives participants the opportunity to actively enhance the lives of others.

Laughter Yoga has the power to change the selfish state of mind to an altruistic state of mind. It has been proven that people who laugh are likely to be more generous and have more empathy than those who don't laugh. This inner spirit of laughter becomes apparent as people develop a state of internal peace: the worries and intense goals that have driven their lives become less important.

These people become aware that true happiness comes from giving unconditional love, caring for others, and sharing with each other. Laughter Yoga inspires members to make the world a better place not only for themselves, but for every one.

Except from: Kataria, M. (2011), *Laugh for no reason*.

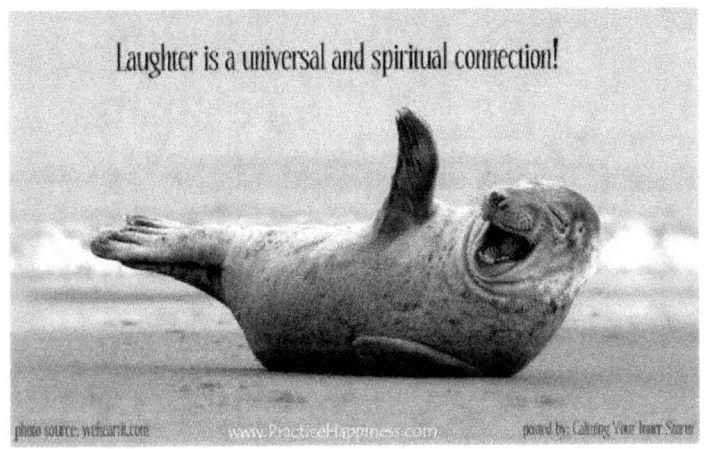

Laughter brings you to reality as it is. The world is a play of God, a cosmic joke. And unless you understand it as a cosmic joke you will never be able to understand the ultimate mystery.

Bhagwan Shree Rajneesh
Indian Spiritual leader

10. SPIRITUAL LAUGHTER

I consider myself a Christian Buddhist mystic. What exactly that means, however, I can't say for sure. Having been raised without religion, I, like many others, turned to Christianity. In 6th grade, my family moved to a small farming community and I was sent to a fundamentalist Christian school. I will never forget my first day. *"Open to John 3:16,"* the teacher said. Her words struck fear in my heart. Having never seen a Bible before, I was beyond lost. Fumbling to find my place, a fellow student grabbed the text from my hands and located the desired page. As she plopped the book loudly on the desk in front of me, all eyes turned my way. Right then and there I vowed that this embarrassment would never happen again: I would figure this religion thing out.

Though my parents knew nothing of my

dilemma or my growing faith, from 6th grade forward, I attended daily Bible classes, prayer groups and weekly services. I was sent to an all girls' Catholic high school and my emersion in religiosity continued. Throughout my college years, I consistently visited churches, often sneaking in mid-day, just to sit quietly in the space. Though I rarely participated in an actual service, I frequently sought comfort and solitude in the confines of an open church.

In college, I took classes in philosophy and Eastern Asian religions. Yet, as the years passed and my adult life unfolded, I slowly deconstructed (and eventually reconstructed) my faith. Marrying an agnostic man, my traditional religiosity had all but vanished.

For better or worse, my children were raised without religion. Though we half-heartedly attended a Presbyterian church, our occasional presence had little effect on anyone. Each child was given a Bible in elementary school, though its introduction was made in the form of a great literary work.

I was married for nearly 18 years and life continued on. My passion for religion remained dormant. Post divorce, however, I was surprised to find myself falling into Buddhism. Words like compassion and detachment began to appear in my vocabulary. Suffering became a choice; expectations and ego dissolved. As I struggled to let go of my marriage and find forgiveness for my ex, the constructs of Buddhism became increasingly attractive.

In the years that followed, I dabbled in all aspects of the spiritual realm, reading the works of John of the Cross, Teresa of Avila, Khalil Gibran, and my beloved, Carolyn Myss. I began to meditate, and once again, to pray, but nothing amazing happened .

Nothing that is, until, in my early 50s, I stumbled into the Laugher Yoga Leader training course at Yogaville. Just as I had progressed from Christianity to Catholicism, and Catholicism to Buddhism; it seems I had passed through Buddhism and fell headlong into laughter.

Henry Miller writes: *"Laughter is the most direct route to God, filling our heads with light as we go..."* And for me, at least, Miller was right.

You may recall from the introduction, I wasn't blessed with a family that laughed. In fact, I grew up being told that only hyenas laugh. My mother, much like Lord Chesterfield, seem to believe that laughter was somehow vulgar and unladylike. Perhaps that is, in part, why my journey into laughter was so liberating.

In re-discovering, or more accurately, finally discovering my laugh, I've learned to let go of my ego. (The ego is unable to laugh at itself and has no choice but to fall into place.) Osho (1985) explains that to laugh at others is egotistic, but to laugh at oneself is to be humble.

Nothing kills the ego like playfulness, like laughter. When you start taking life as fun, the ego has to die, it cannot exist anymore. -Osho

And sure enough, in beginning to laugh at myself, I became lighter. My attachment to ego decreased. (Granted, I still have a long way to go on this one!) Ironically, as my ego quieted, I seemed to step into myself. I became louder. I spoke up - my voice, my breath, my laugh - everything about me began to "speak up." Having less fear of judgment, less concern for social norms, I found myself happier, finding humor in the craziest places.

As I deconstructed Buddhism - or more accurately, deconstructed my ego, I was left with laughter - my laughter, the vibration which linked me to God.

Your laugh is your personal vibration in this world. Let's face it, no one shares your exact laugh. Just as your fingerprint or genetic make up is uniquely you, so too is your laugh. (And to think that the Gods have given me, an introvert raised to fit in, such a loud *hurp, hurp, hurp, exhale* vibration is pretty funny in and of itself.)

Many spiritual traditions seek to understand and internalize the nature of God. They strive to dismantle the ego, develop compassion and understand both the higher SELF and the ego self. It is well known that laughter can shorten the distance between our self and others, but far fewer people realize that intentional laughter can also shorten the distance between the higher SELF and ego self.

Yogic laughter, ironically provides a way for us to lose ourselves in order to find our higher selves. In other words, a regular laughter practice creates space for the true self to emerge as we let go of our seriousness, anxiety and ego.

But is dissolving ego enough to keep you laughing? Buddha wrote:

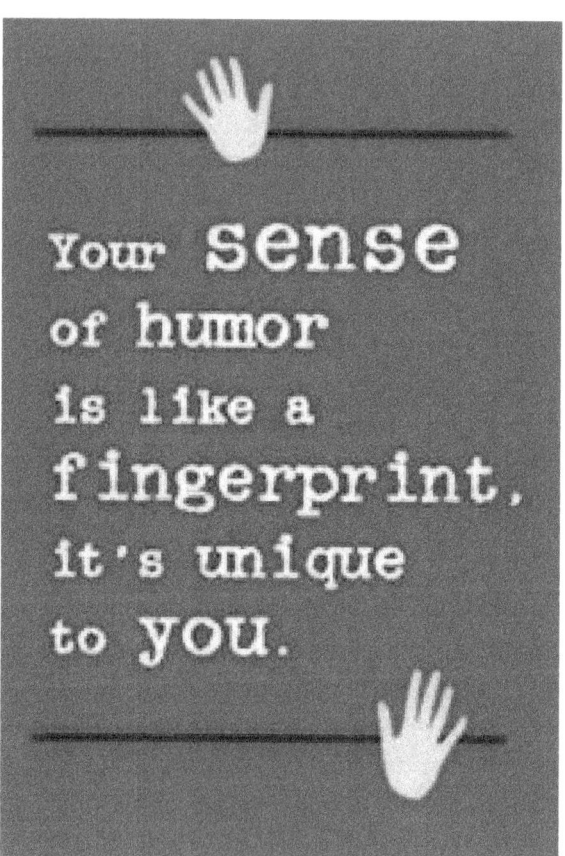

"When you realize how perfect everything is you will tilt your head back and laugh at the sky."

Osho seems to agree:

"The whole play of existence is so beautiful that laughter can be the only response to it. Only laughter can be the real prayer, gratitude."

Even Anne Lamott is in on the secret, stating that:

"Laughter is carbonated holiness."

Was that what happened to me? Was I simply releasing some ego? Had I realized how perfect everything is? How beautiful? No. In fact, I would venture to say that what led me to laughter was exactly the opposite. I'd realized how deeply flawed my logic had been; how silly, how imperfect - beautifully imperfect, perhaps, but imperfect nonetheless. I'd set out to understand, constrain and somehow control the force and nature of God. How silly was that?

Dr. Kataria describes two paths into spirituality. He writes:

"There are two ways we can become spiritual. One is religious, meditation, yoga. I believe that's long and very

difficult. It takes years to become spiritual. Another way you can become spiritual is to raise your spirits: Raise someone else's spirits... You don't need to spend hours in temple chanting mantras. You play like a child. Flow from your heart with your love, compassion, appreciation, forgiveness. You are spiritual."

WHAT SOAP IS TO THE BODY, LAUGHTER IS TO THE SOUL.

QUOTEHD.COM

Yiddish Proverb

To date, Zen Buddhism is the only religion that has accepted laughter as a form of prayer. In Zen monasteries the monks laugh at themselves each morning before they rise and each evening before they retire.

In fact, when Bodhidharma, a 5th or 6th century Buddhist monk who is credited with founding Chan Buddhism, became enlightened, he is said to have started laughing and never stopped. When asked why he was laughing, Bodhidharma replied;

"I go on laughing because what I have been searching for was always within me. I was such an idiot; I cannot believe that for so many lives I have been searching for something with was already within me. In fact, the searcher was the sought; the seeker was the goal."

"There was no other goal except myself to be found. And when I see others doing the same, I cannot stop laughing at the ridiculousness of the whole search, of the whole spirituality." (Osho 1987).

In truth, I feel a little bit like Bodhidharma - minus the 13 years spent meditating in a cave and obtaining enlightenment, of course. But for better or worse, I too laugh at myself and my ego on a daily basis.

I laugh because I to try to control the uncontrollable, I try to understand that which cannot be understood. I pretend I'm not human - not fallible. When I'm weak, I pretend to be strong. And yet when I'm strong, I pretend to be weak. How funny is that? I pretend not to be mad, not to be nervous. I often pretend not to care when I do, and occasionally I pretend to care when I don't. I am hysterical, ridiculous.

We are all ridiculous. We rush around achieving and obtaining - only to die unable to take any of it with us. We create importance; we create meaning. As if the whole of life - the entirety of the universe depended on our upcoming sale, presentation, vacation, grade, job, appearance or even our hairstyle. I mean come on, how funny is that?

Never be afraid to laugh at yourself. After all, you could be missing out on the joke of the century.

meetville.com

Dame Edna Everage

And the irony of this lifetime continues. We are born, as infants, dependent on others for care. Then, throughout the entirety of our lives, we move away from that state. We grow, we thrive, we achieve, we seek, only to eventually arrive right back were we started! And if, by chance, we are blessed to die before the cycle is complete, we are said to have died too soon! How funny is that? Die with your senses intact, your mind sharp, and your body active, whether you're 40, 50, 60, or even 70, and we say you have died too soon, too young; how unfortunate, how sad. Yet live until you return to a child-like state; live long enough to arrive exactly where you had started and the cycle is complete. You've succeeded. Congratulations on a life well lived!

Osho writes:

"Laughter brings you to the earth, brings you down from your stupid idea of being holier - than- thou. Laughter brings you to reality as it is. The world is a play of God: A cosmic joke. Unless you understand it is a cosmic joke you will never be able to understand the ultimate mystery."

I cannot help but to agree. How can we not laugh? How can we not see the humor in humanity? We are serious - so serious. We're taught to be serious; taught to suppress our laughter: To laugh at the correct decibel for the correct amount of time.

Seriousness is thought to be a sign of respect, a badge of honor. Work and worry, success and achievement, are honored above laughter and play. Yet where does it get us? Right back to where we started! We struggle and rush our lives away, only to arrive exactly where we started. Tell me that's not funny.

> I think that wherever your journey takes you, there are new gods waiting there, with divine patience - and laughter.
>
> Susan M. Watkins

As demonstrated earlier, some level of seriousness and control is necessary for society to function. But how far should it go?

Voltaire, a late 17th / early 18th century writer, historian, and philosopher wrote: *"God is a comedian playing to an audience too afraid to laugh."*

Is he right? Have we missed God by forgetting how to laugh? But Voltaire lived and died in France, over 200 years ago. What progress have we made? Sadly perhaps, not nearly enough.

Osho (1985) states that: *"seriousness is a sin - a disease. Seriousness starts wars. Murders are committed by serious people; suicide is the act of a serious person."* Osho goes on to suggest that throughout history, the king's court has needed a fool. Without the presence of a court jester seriousness would spread uncontrollably. In short, these fools provide the necessary balance for seriousness. They provide levity and encouraged new ways of thinking.

Jean Houston writes: *"At the height of laughter, the universe is flung into a kaleidoscope of new possibilities."* Perhaps medieval kings were on to something.

Yet the need for humor and laughter was recognized long before kings and court jesters arrived on the scene. In fact, one of the world's earliest printed texts: A Hindu religious scripture *Hymn from the Rig Veda*, (c. 1200–900 BC), refers to *"fun making for the creation of laughter"* Though our court jesters have been replaced by comedians, romantic comedies, and yes, even online cat videos, the desire for balance between humor and seriousness is one we still seek today.

Most people accept that humor and laughter are central to the human condition, yet many baulk at the idea that having a sense of humor is, in fact, a necessary spiritual trait.

Steve Brown in his book: *Approaching God: Accepting the Invitation to Stand in the Presence of God writes:*

> *"If there is no laughter, Jesus has gone somewhere else. If there is no joy and freedom, it is not a church: it is simply a crowd of melancholy people basking in a religious neurosis. If there is no celebration, there is no real worship."*

Osho proposes that we are drawn to images of Christ suffering because we too are suffering; that we too have crosses and burdens to bare. But is this suffering necessary? Laughter and joy are readily available to us. Our inner-child is always with us; waiting to be rediscovered.

Personally, I have come to believe that laughter is the vibration of God, or at least as close as we can get to it during our physical incarnation. Laughter is the voice and natural expression of God. I believe we are never closer to God than when we are laughing.

Now before you judge me as crazy: Think

about it. Laughter heals. It provides pain relief, draws people together, eliminates anger, and is always available to us. Laugh and reap the rewards; don't laugh and continue to suffer. Laughter doesn't chase after you, it doesn't long to hear your story, or even consider you all that unique: Laughter simply is:

Osho writes:

"If you become silent after your laughter,
one day you will hear God also laughing,
you will hear the whole existence laughing
-- trees and stones and stars with you."

Children come into this world armed with joy, laughter, play and trust. Joy is our natural state. Joy is the state in which we are closest to God. In joy there is innocence. In joy there is connection. In joy there is love. And yes, deep in the heart of joy we find God.

Alan Watts writes of a Roman priest who states: "I always laugh at the altar, be it Christian, Hindu, or Buddhist, because real religion is the transformation of anxiety into laughter." I have to agree. Not about laughing at the alter of other religions, but rather the idea that religion serves to transform anxiety.

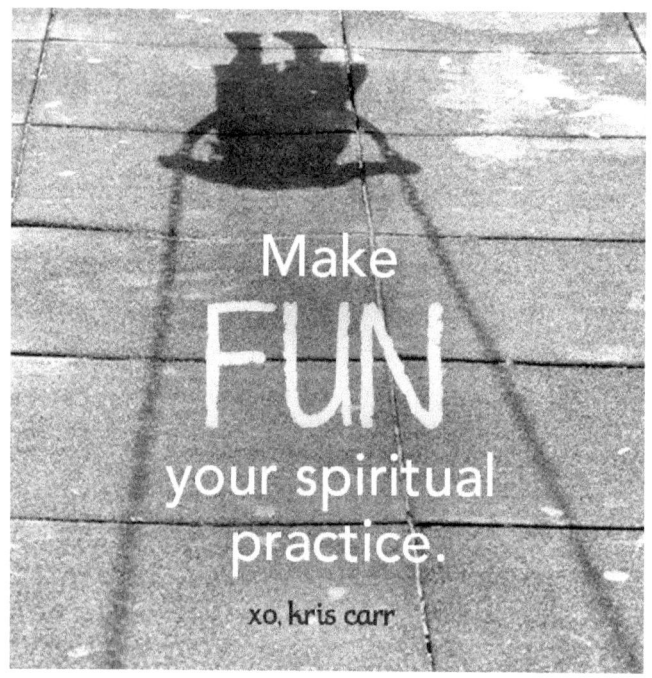

Make
FUN
your spiritual
practice.
xo, kris carr

11. LAUGHING ALONE: HOW FUNNY IS THAT?

True confession: I laugh when I drive. In fact, sometimes, I laugh so hard I can hardly see straight. Why? No reason. I've simply decided to laugh

Let's face it - the world is a serious place! Between work stress, family stress, advertising and marketing guilt, laughter is a welcome relief. Not to mention the fact that the health benefits make it well worth the exercise!

So even as a laughter yoga teacher, I make time to exercise my laugh. Sometimes I laugh when I'm running, but mostly I laugh in the car. More specifically, I laugh each time I cross a bridge - which living in the Tidewater area of Virginia happens a lot!

Truth be told, I'm scared of bridges - pretty much all bridges, but a few in particular terrify me. Yet teaching laughter yoga in Williamsburg, Richmond and Hampton, I cross one of the worst of these bridges on a weekly basis. This bridge is long - it's high and it goes on forever! Yet each time my car rolls up and over this wretched expanse, I laugh - each time - every time - without exception. I guess bursting into laughter, is better than having a panic attack and bursting into tears, which honestly, was the previous choice.

Little did I know, however, that it would be this practice, this bridge, which would change my life and trigger my return to Yogaville. You see, I'd promised myself that I'd laugh each and every time I crossed the bridge and I had - each day, each week, for about 6 months. But one June day, I was singing along to the radio and simply forgot to laugh. As my mid-bridge anxiety rose, it hit me like a ton of bricks, I wasn't laughing on the bridge. In fact, I wasn't laughing at home either.

Having a physical stimulus or an environmental cue, can be a huge asset to your laughter practice. When I realized that I'd forgotten to laugh on the bridge, I simultaneously realized that I was losing the passion for laughter in all aspects of my life. I promptly went back to Yogaville to repeat the Laughter Yoga Leader certification course. Had I not developed this habit, I may have remained unaware of the subtle ways in which I had slowly shifted back to seriousness.

Laughing alone can be tricky, but to reap the full psychological, social, and physical benefits of laughter, you will need to establish a personal practice.

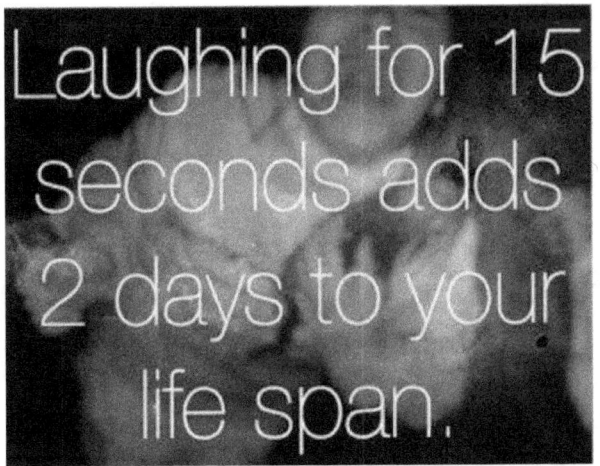

Like the Zen monks, Dr. Kataria encourages his students to laugh for 10 to 15 minutes each morning. This style of laughter is often referred to as a laughing meditation. It is a dynamic practice which encourages the individual to focus on the sound of his or her own laughter; much like one would focus on the breath or a mantra in a more traditional meditation. Arising each morning in laughter awakens the breath and sets the tone for the day.

Yet, there are a variety of other ways to bring more laughter into your life. Perhaps you, like me, will choose to laugh in the car. Laughing in the shower is also popular. Want to take it up a notch? Laugh when you look at yourself in the mirror.

Whatever practice you choose, the key is to be consistent. Be committed. Join a "laughter gym." Develop a routine and continue to practice. Just as you would lift weights or run on a treadmill, laughter yoga is an exercise. And like all forms of exercise, the more you do it, the easier it becomes.

The following pages offer a few tips from Dr. Kataria to help get and keep you laughing. But remember: There is no right or wrong in laughter. There's no failure; no judgment. As soon as you are willing, your life will begin to change.

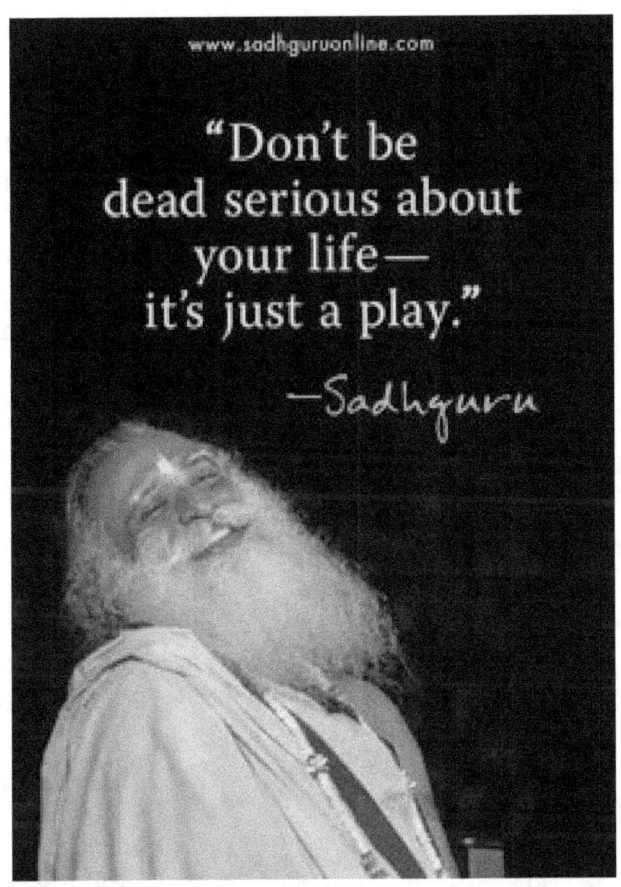

TIPS TO KEEP YOU LAUGHING

Be Willing:

It is very important to have the willingness to laugh. Try to put feeling into your laughter. Fully express yourself and release suppressed emotions.

Have a Positive Self-Dialogue:

Don't judge the quality of your laughter. Don't tell yourself it's not real or spontaneous laughter. You are choosing to laugh and play as a form of an exercise. You're seeking proven health benefits and increasing the oxygen in your body. Notice, appreciate, and give yourself a pat on the back each time you laugh.

Commit for 40-Days:

If you continue to do laughter yoga alone for 40 days it will become a habit. The brain develops new circuits and the act becomes a part of your unconscious mind. So set a goal for 40 days!

By laughing alone for 40 days your brain will

develop new neuronal connections to produce neuropeptides and happiness hormones. In the language of neuro-linguistic programing, this is called developing an "ANCHOR". By physically performing a joyful anchor action, the mind experiences the emotion of joy (complete with the chemical reactions it triggers). In that way, our body and mind can be trained to laugh at will.

Life is too short
to be serious all the time....
So, if you can't laugh
at yourself,
Call me.... I'll laugh at YOU.

Remember: Laughter Is All About Playfulness:

As laughter is all about cultivating childlike playfulness, it comes straight from the body and does not make use of any intellectual capacity of the brain. Even alone, you can devise methods and exercises that help induce laughter in the body. Laughing alone is the easiest way to overcome psychological barriers and inhibitions.

Once you learn to play, laughter is a natural outcome.

Remember: Every Person Is Different:

There is no one correct way of laughing. People can develop their own comfort zone with different sounds and gestures and different postures that facilitate laughing alone. Create your own exercises and develop new ideas to discover what works best for you.

TIPS TO GET YOU STARTED

Open Your Mouth Wide

Relax your jaw. Each time you do laughter exercises; open your mouth a bit wider to enable laughter from the belly. If your mouth is tightly closed, laughter will come from the throat or the upper chest.

Wear Loose Clothing

Wear loose and comfortable clothes that allow you to breath and laugh freely. Pants should fall below the naval and should not obstruct the abdominal movements. Avoid tight belts.

Duration and Ideal Time

Aim for 15 minutes a day of yogic breathing and laughter exercises, with short breaks of relaxation. Begin with 5 or 10 minutes and gradually increase the duration.

Laughing alone should be practiced the first thing in the morning as it will set your mood for the day. Begin with some warming up and breathing exercises. This will help facilitate laughter.

If you don't feel like laughing early in the morning, laughing anytime of day will boost your energy levels.

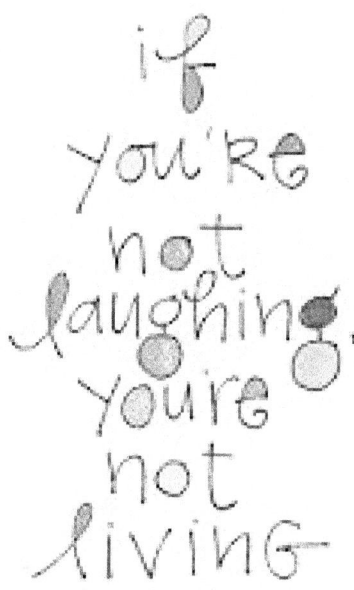

Warm Up Exercises

Before you start, do some warm up exercises: Ho Ho Ha Ha, practice gibberish, tongue swirling and a few very good very good yeahs. These are great physical expressions of joy, which will help set the stage.

These exercises will be a lot more fun if you do them in front of a mirror. Change the pitch and tone of your voice to find your comfort levels. Begin gently or quietly and gradually increase the intensity as you get more comfortable.

Fake It Until You Make It

- The slogan of all laughter yoga clubs is, 'fake it until you make it'. This is based on a scientific fact that even if you are faking a particular emotion, the body cannot differentiate between real and fake emotions.

- Try faking laughter by making different sounds of laughter Ha ha ha He he he he Ho ho ho.... and keep playing with these exercises. It is a kind of silliness. You will discover that you start laughing genuinely while hearing the absurd sounds of your own laughter.

- Keep trying different ways of faking laughter sounds and you'll find some of them affordable and amusing. Stick to them and practice it more and more.

Initially fake laughter may seem awkward, but with practice your body will become conditioned and the moment you start faking laughter it will turn to real laughter very quickly.

Sound of Laughter

As children, we shout and scream to express ourselves, but as adults we learn to control the pitch and tone of our voice. As a result, we are not able to express our feelings to the fullest. The freedom and expression of the voice effects the freedom of emotions in the mind and vice versa. This is the reason that everyone has a distinct sound of laughter. The way one laughs is a signature of one's character.

Laughing Alone In The Bathroom

The bathroom provides a place for privacy and safety. You can be as funny as you want to and have no fear of anyone watching. Regularly laughing in the shower gets programmed into the body. The moment you turn on the water, you will start laughing automatically. This is the benefit of repeating any activity and combining physical behavior and with it.

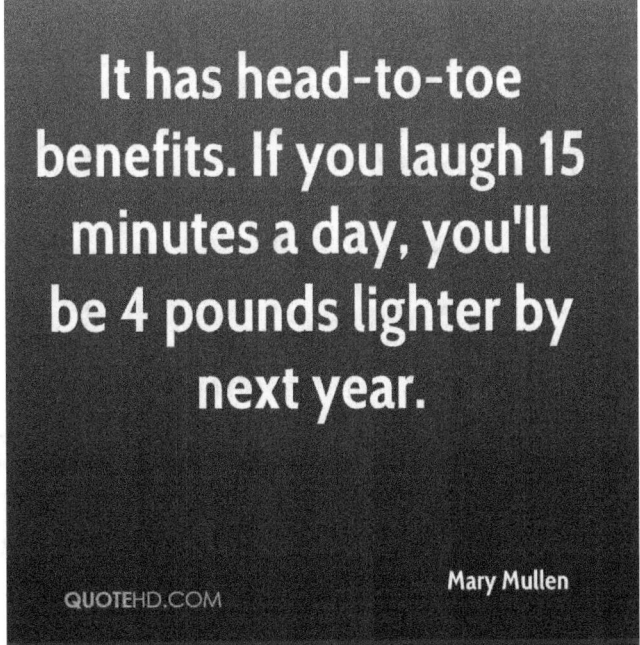

It has head-to-toe benefits. If you laugh 15 minutes a day, you'll be 4 pounds lighter by next year.

Mary Mullen

QUOTEHD.COM

Walking and Laughing

While walking alone, you can find a safe place and laugh at the top of your voice and experience the feeling of freedom.

Laughing in The Car

Laughing alone can be very effective while driving, especially with traffic and other daily irritants. Instead of losing patience, laugh away these situations. You can do the *ho ho ha ha* exercise without any sound. It all depends upon your level of comfort as you might be aware of other people watching you laughing. You can also pick up your mobile phone and pretend to laugh for a few minutes.

Laugh at Yourself - Ha Ha Mantra

Laughing at yourself is not about degradation, but is a gentle reminder that life is too serious. To keep your spirits high, instead of laughing you can just say haaaaa haaaaa haaaaa few times and it will make you feel better. I always use this Ha Ha Mantra when I mess up something or drop food on my shirt or when something falls from my hands.

Ha Ha Mantra For Free Floating Hostilities

Our lives are flooded with innumerable situations that give rise to irritability and stress. We call them *'free floating hostilities'* as they are freely available everywhere. These infuriating situations bring a big change in your temperament and attitude.

The best substitute for these hostilities is the Ha Ha Manta. Every time you find such a frustrating situation remember to *haaaaaaa haaaaaaa haaaaaa.*

Laughing With Household Chores

You can laugh while doing repetitive household chores like washing dishes, mopping the floor, vacuuming, cleaning, hanging clothes, cleaning windows and many others. This is not a loud laughter, but a gentle giggle which will help to change your perspective towards mundane chores and will make them less daunting.

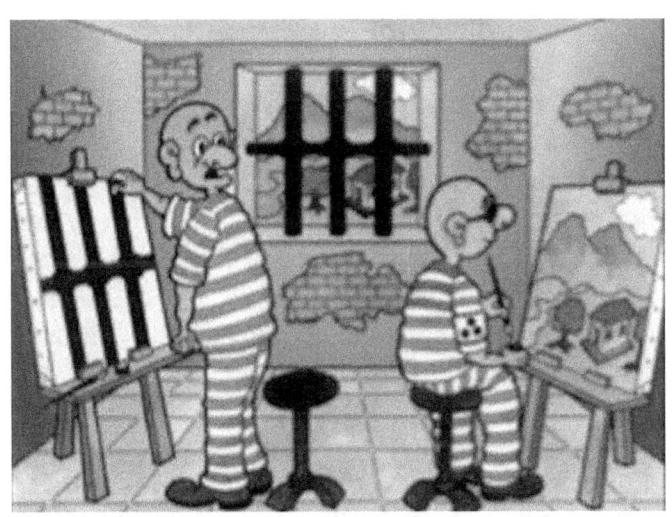

12. THE TRANSFORMATIVE POWER OF INTENTIONAL LAUGHTER

When I went home for Christmas, I was laughing. In fact, I was laughing a lot. My mom wasn't happy. Truth be told, I'm guessing my children and sister were also a bit confused. Only seeing each other for brief periods of time scattered throughout the year, I doubt that anyone fully understood the path I'd been on. It's one thing to say I teach laughter yoga... maybe chucking a bit more on the phone than usual, it's quite another to sound like a hyena at Christmas dinner.

But there I was laughing, much to my mother's chagrin. There was no hiding it: Laughter yoga had changed me. And it will change you as well.

> **When You Laugh,**
> **You Change,**
> **When You Change,**
> **The Whole**
> **World Changes**
>
> Dr. Madan Kataria
>
> www.laughteryoga.org

When I first arrived in Yogaville, I thought our teacher, Bharta Wingham was crazy, but the light of his soul filled the room. When I studied with Dr. Madan Kataria, the founder of the laughter yoga movement, a year later, I had a similar experience. Being an Indian medical doctor, Dr. Kataria's mannerisms, are far more reserved, but like Bharta, his spirit filled the room. Both men felt light - lighthearted - almost as if they were vibrating in laughter.

Though I'm guessing I have years to go to catch up to them on that front, practicing intentional laughter has changed me.

Ironically, in learning to laugh, I found parts of myself I never knew existed. I became louder... my laugh is loud! (much to my mother's chagrin). And I seem to burst out laughing at the slightest stimulus.   Far from a quiet *ha ha* or lady-like giggle when something funny happens - I'm all in! *Hurp, hurp hurp, exhale. Hurp hurp hurp, exhale.* I can't help it, can't stop it, and honestly, I wouldn't want too.

My laugh, crazy as it is, makes others laugh, something I now see as a tremendous blessing. After years of searching for a way to contribute to society, laughter yoga has proven the perfect venue. As an introvert, I bring something others don't. I understand that laughter can be frightening; that finding your laugh is not always easy. I've chosen to work with individuals who also struggle to laugh: cancer patients, those working to overcome a chronic illness or battling obesity.

But more importantly perhaps, bringing more laughter into my life has altered my spiritual journey.   My ego, though still present in all aspects of my life, is no longer in the driver's seat. I don't hold on to mistakes and I don't react to the little dramas of daily life.

In fact, when the plumber informed me that the water main had broken under my house, I simply burst out laughing! The look on his face was priceless: a mixture of confusion and fear. When I finally stopped, he replied that he'd never seen a homeowner have that reaction before. Something I took as a complement, although I'm not sure that was his intent.

Laughter Yoga has also brought people into my life. Great people. We laugh and play, dance and act silly. I speak up now. I breath deeply and annunciate clearly. I also take risks. Being able to laugh at myself has eradicated the fear of anyone else laughing at me. If I'm already laughing, no one can laugh at me, they're simply joining me. Once, while giving a talk at NASA, for example, I completely forgot what to say. Standing on the stage with all eyes on me, I suddenly had nothing - not a thought in my head. Fortunately, the talk was about laughter - learning to laugh at yourself and bringing more laughter into your life. So what did I do? I laughed! In fact, I laughed a lot. The audience laughed. I freely admitted that I'd lost my train of thought, and we moved quickly into a laughter yoga exercise called: *I forgot to laugh.* As soon as the tension lifted, I continued the lecture with ease.

SHE
IS CLOTHED IN
STRENGTH
AND
DIGNITY,
AND SHE
LAUGHS
WITHOUT FEAR
OF THE FUTURE.

In the presence of laughter, seriousness dissipates. It has no choice. When there is light, the darkness retreats. Where there is laughter, anxiety and fear diminish. Laughter brings people together. It humanizes us.

Victor Borge writes: *"Laughter is the shortest distance between people."* And I couldn't agree more.

Learning to laugh in my early 50s, however, has left me with one regret. I'm sorry that I failed to raise my children in an environment of laughter. I wish now that I had given them the opportunity to more fully embrace the joy of being a child. We laughed, of course, but with constraint. Outside voices were meant to be used outside, and outside only. Their laughter, although allowed and encouraged, was typically classified as appropriate or inappropriate, depending on the situation, and it was always practiced with control. If I had it to do over again, I would change that. But perhaps that's what grandchildren are for.

So for now, I will continue my journey into laughter, anxious to see where it leads. It is my hope, of course, that others will follow. That I too will someday appear both enlightened and insane to an unsuspecting student.

In the meantime, however, I reckon I'll continue to sound like a hyena, much to my mother's chagrin.

Hurp hurp hurp, exhale.
Hurp hurp hurp, exhale.

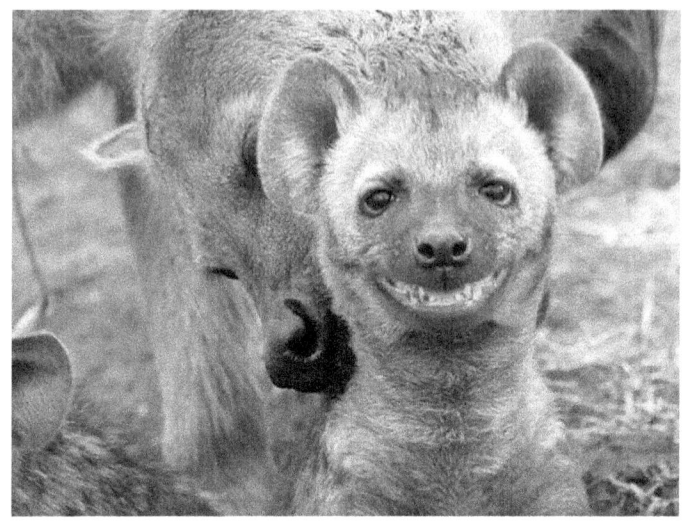

Sorry Mom...

In love and laughter,

Jessica

she
laughs
proverbs 31:25

REFERENCES

Altucher, James (2014), retrieved on July 1, 2015
From
http://www.jamesaltucher.com/2014/04/w
hat-happened-to-all-

Berk, L.S. et al., (1989), Neuroendocrine and
stress hormone changes during mirthful
laughter. Retrieved on August 1,2015 from:
http://www.ncbi.nlm.nih.gov/pubmed/2556
917

Cousins, Norman. (1979). *Anatomy of an Illness.*
New York: Norton.

Cousins, N. (1990). *Head first: The biology of hope
and the human spirit.* Penguin Books, NY, NY.

Elias, M. (March 13, 2007), Study links sense of
     humor, survival. *USA Today.*
     retrieved   on   Aug   2,   2015   from
     http://usatoday30.usatoday.com/tech/scienc
     e/discoveries/2007-03-13-humor-
     study_N.htm

Foley E, Matheis R, Schaefer C. , (2002). Effect of
     forced laughter on mood. *Psychol Rep.* 90
     (1):184.

Fry, W. (1994). The biology of humor.
     International Journal of Humor Research 7,
     111-126.

Kataria, M. (2011), *Laugh for no reason.* Madhuri
     International: Mumbai India.

Mayo Clinic (June 20, 2013) retrieved from
     http://www.cbsnews.com/news/study-
     shows-70-percent-of-americans-take-
     prescription-drugs/

Nasr, SJ., (2013). No laughing matter: Laughter is
     good psychiatric medicine, *Current
     Psychiatry*, August;12(8):20-25.

U.K.A. (2004, Aug). Study Confirms Belief that
Laughter is the Best Medicine. *AORN Journal.*
Denver: Colorado.

Osho (1987) *Life, love, laughter: Celebrating your existence.* St. Martin's Griffin, NY, NY.

Young R. & Redford Young, S., (2002). *The Ph Miracle.* Warner Books. NY.

Sebastian, S. (July, 2003) retrieved on Aug 9, 2015,from: http://articles.chicagotribune.com/2003-07-29/features/0307290281_1_laughing-40th-anniversary-village

Srini, G (2010). Retrieved on July, 17, 2015 from: https://jnanagni.wordpress.com/2010/09/18/pleasure-and-pain-heat-and-cold-bhagavad-gita-2-14-15/

Semenza G. L. (2009). Defining the role of hypoxia-inducible factor 1 in cancer biology and therapeutics. Oncogene retrieved on September 4, 2015 from: http://www.nature.com/onc/journal/v29/n5/abs/onc2009441a.html

Thom, M. & Wright, M. (2013), *Change your body: Is your body acidic or alkaline*? ebook: Retrieved on Nov. 9, 2015 from https://books.google.com/books?id=n4iZAgAAQBAJ&pg=PT103&lpg=PT103&dq=laughter+body+alkaline&source=bl&ots=dW3A_eTR

NR&sig=J94EulQOVyMOleuFJSZpRkJ5nmk&h
l=en&sa=X&ved=0CDEQ6AEwA2oVChMI7uvI
oruEyQIVVvBjCh2QOwSX#v=onepage&q=lau
ghter%20body%20alkaline&f=false.

Wingham, B. (ND) *Laugha yoga: Combining the joy of laughter with the bliss of yoga.* Satchidananda Ashram, Yogaville, VA.

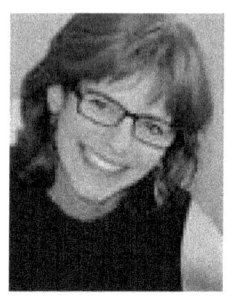

ABOUT THE AUTHOR

Jessica Lloyd, PhD, RN is a certified laughter yoga teacher and a laughter ambassador. She is the author of several books including: *Embracing Impermanence*, Worth A Shot Gallery's *Rules to Live By* and *Attitude is Everything*.

Jessica is currently teaching laughter yoga in the Williamsburg, Richmond, and the Tidewater area of Virginia. She is the owner and chief laughter yogi at The Laughing Buddha, an interactive healing arts gallery, featuring laughter yoga, yoga, meditation, and qigong.

THE LAUGHING BUDDHA

The Laughing Buddha is an interactive healing arts gallery promoting healing, health and happiness through laughter. We are a membership based community offering classes in laughter yoga, yoga, meditation and qigong as well as a variety of health and healing work-shops.

Laughter yoga is offered once a week at The Laughing Buddha as a free, or donation based, class with all proceeds being donated to Save the Chimps, a chimpanzee sanctuary.

We are located on Bypass Rd. in Williamsburg, VA. Please visit our website or find us on Facebook, for more information or to view our programing.

www.the-laughing-buddha.com

facebook.com/tlbuddha